# Progress against Heart Disease

# Progress against Heart Disease

## FRED C. PAMPEL AND SETH PAULEY

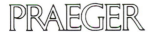 PRAEGER

**Westport, Connecticut**
**London**

**Library of Congress Cataloging-in-Publication Data**

Pampel, Fred C.
    Progress against heart disease / Fred C. Pampel and Seth Pauley.
        p. cm.
    Includes bibliographical references.
    ISBN 0–275–98151–7 (alk. paper)
    1. Heart—Diseases—Popular works.
    [DNLM: 1. Heart Diseases—prevention & control. 2. Heart Diseases—diagnosis. 3. Life
Style. WG 210 P185p 2004] I. Pauley, Seth. II. Title.
RC672.P35   2004
616.1′2—dc22          2004008832

British Library Cataloguing in Publication Data is available.

Library of Congress Catalog Card Number: 2004008832
ISBN: 0–275–98151–7

First published in 2004

Praeger Publishers, 88 Post Road West, Westport, CT 06881
An imprint of Greenwood Publishing Group, Inc.
www.praeger.com

Printed in the United States of America

The paper used in this book complies with the
Permanent Paper Standard issued by the National
Information Standards Organization (Z39.48–1984).

10  9  8  7  6  5  4  3  2  1

# Contents

# Figures

# PART I

## Changes

# CHAPTER 1

# Counting the Lives Saved

In 1978, the same year he won election to the first of his five terms as a Wyoming congressman, Dick Cheney had his first heart attack. He suffered another attack in 1984 and then a third in 1988 at age 47, but heart bypass surgery stabilized his condition until November 2000. While running for vice president, he experienced chest pains, and doctors inserted a coronary stent to prop open a narrow artery. In March 2001, now Vice President Cheney entered a Washington, D.C., hospital with chest pains and underwent a procedure to reopen the blocked artery. Just a few months later, he had a device implanted to monitor and, if necessary, slow his heart rhythm. After the surgery, the doctors said his prognosis was "terrific." Now over age 60 and with a 23-year history of heart problems, Vice President Cheney remains fully active in his duties. He sticks faithfully to his diet and exercises almost daily on his stationary bike.[1]

In January 2000, *Late Show* host David Letterman announced to guest Regis Philbin and the audience that he planned to undergo some heart tests. He said he had very high cholesterol ("Its borderline . . . 680," he joked) and a lifestyle not well suited to a healthy heart. Moreover, his father had a heart attack at age 36 and died of a coronary attack at age 57 in 1973. After the test showed blockages in his arteries, Letterman underwent emergency quintuple bypass surgery.[2] The procedure was a complete success, allowing the host to return to the show a few weeks later. Whatever problems led to the blockages, Letterman is doing well. He now jogs regularly, has lost weight, follows a low-fat diet, and continues to host his late-night show.

In 1957 at age 40, Nathan Pritikin discovered he had a seriously high blood cholesterol level of 300. An abnormal electrocardiogram stress test later confirmed the worst—substantial coronary heart disease. To avoid drugs, surgery, or a life of inactivity, he changed his diet to eliminate nearly all fat and began walking and then jogging for an hour a day. His cholesterol plummeted to below 125, and another electrocardiogram stress test in the mid-1960s proved completely normal. His lifestyle change seemed not just to control but actually to eliminate his heart disease. Eventually, he wrote best-selling books and opened a popular California spa that promised to improve health with exercise and an extremely low fat diet. He died in 1985 at age 69, some 28 years after his first diagnosis, from causes unrelated to heart disease. An autopsy indicated he had an "absolutely remarkable" absence of cholesterol fatty deposits and calcification in his coronary arteries.[3]

These stories illustrate both the risks of heart disease and the promise in dealing with the risks. The risks of heart disease afflict the famous as well as the ordinary. The promise shows in the potential that changes in lifestyle and medical treatment have to allow people to live full lives despite having heart disease. Although people often know that heart disease is the number-one killer in the United States, they seldom realize the enormous progress made in preventing and treating the disease. The progress represents a remarkable story of scientific discovery and social change in lifestyles. To give a few examples, the lives of Americans have been extended by the

- development of machines to keep pumping blood while doing surgery on the heart,
- widespread use of emergency care to keep victims of cardiac arrest alive,
- invention of anticlotting and cholesterol drugs to prevent heart attacks,
- reliance on routine diagnostic tests to identify heart problems early,
- dramatic decline of cigarette use since the 1960s, and
- adoption of better diets and exercise activities.

As a result of this progress, the life expectancy of Americans, according to the most recently released figures, reached an all-time high in 2001 of 79.8 years for women, 74.4 years for men, and 77.2 years for men and women combined.[4] And declining mortality from diseases of the heart contributes significantly to this record-high life expectancy. Consideration of the extent of the problem of heart disease in the United States must therefore be balanced by consideration of the progress made against the problem in the last several decades.

## EXTENT OF THE PROBLEM

Heart disease affects large parts of the population. In the United States in the year 2000, 12.6 million Americans had coronary heart disease, 4.8

million had problems of a weakened heart, and 2.0 million had faulty heart rhythms. These problems resulted in 650,000 people who had their first heart attack in 2000, 450,000 who had a recurrent heart attack, and 550,000 who experienced heart failure.[5]

Not surprisingly, heart disease is the number-one killer of Americans. In 2000, 709,894 Americans died of heart disease (29.5 percent of all deaths). The number exceeds the 551,833 deaths from cancer and the 166,028 deaths from strokes.[6] The problem similarly harms members of nearly all race and ethnic groups: heart disease tops other causes of death among whites, blacks, Hispanics, Native Americans, and Asian men. Only Asian women, who have more deaths from cancer than heart disease, deviate from the general pattern.

The problem appears most serious among men but affects millions of women as well. Men experience heart problems at younger ages than women, in large part because estrogen in premenopausal women offers some protection against heart disease. Yet, with such protection ending after menopause, heart disease becomes the number-one killer among both women and men. By age 60, for example, 25 percent of both men and women die of heart disease.[7]

Those who live with heart problems face a serious chronic health condition that often limits daily activities. Only arthritis and back and neck conditions do more than heart disease to disrupt the ability to perform normal tasks of life. The economic costs of heart disease also illustrate the gravity of the problem. Annual expenditures for health care and for lost productivity from heart disease reached 214 billion dollars in 2002.[8] Most of the direct costs come from hospital care, but costs for nursing-home care, physician services, and prescription drugs add substantially to the total. Counting the pain and anxiety faced by those with heart disease further adds to the economic costs.

## PROGRESS IN RECENT DECADES

Things look much better when viewed not in isolation but in comparison to previous decades. The trends over time reveal a substantial, persistent, and remarkable decline in deaths from heart disease. Figure 1.1 shows the age-adjusted death rates of men and women from diseases of the heart over the years 1955 to 1998. After a peak in the late 1960s, the death rates have decreased almost every year since then.

A simple calculation gives a sense of the enormous change implied by the rates shown in figure 1.1. The major type of heart disease—coronary artery disease—accounted for 514,000 deaths in 2000. However, it would have caused 1,329,000 deaths if the rate had remained at its 1968 peak.[9] We tend to take this progress for granted, but if put in the form of a headline—815,000 LIVES SAVED!—it would rightly gain much more at-

**Figure 1.1**
**Heart Disease Mortality Rates, 1955–1998**

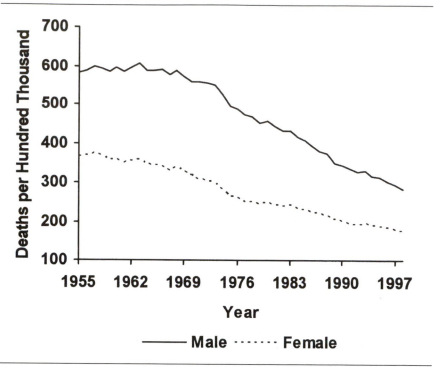

*Source:* World Health Organization, *World Health Statistics Annual* (Geneva, Switzerland: World Health Organization, 1996 and earlier years), http://www.who.int/whosis. (Age-adjusted rates.)

tention. Summing the lives saved for each year since 1968 makes the figure even larger. Based on a projection from zero lives saved in 1968 to the 815,000 lives saved in 1998, the full 31-year time span shows more than *13 million lives saved* due to the lower mortality rates from heart disease.

These lives saved are not limited to the very old, who would die soon of other causes anyway. To the contrary, heart disease mortality has fallen faster among the young and middle-aged than the old.[10] Lowering premature mortality has shifted death from heart disease to the older ages. With family members, friends, coworkers, and neighbors living longer, few of us have not benefited in some way from these trends.

In historical perspective, this is a stunning change. In 1900, heart disease was the fourth most common cause of death in the United States, after pneumonia, tuberculosis, and diarrheal disease. By 1910, it had reached first place in large part because of the decline in deaths from the other infectious diseases. But beginning in 1920, the rate of heart disease mortality began a 30- to 40-year climb. By midcentury, heart disease accounted for more than a third of all deaths. After World War II, the nation addressed this epidemic with major research and public health efforts. The National Heart Institute was created to fund research, the American Heart Association aided with a national campaign to reduce risk factors, and the surgeon general's report warned the public of the risks of cigarette smoking for heart disease (as well as lung cancer, respiratory disease, and a variety of other problems). By the end of the 1960s, heart disease mortality began to fall and has continued the downward trajectory since then.

The decline of heart disease represents one of the most important public health achievements of the twentieth century. As Professor Eugene Braunwald stated in the prestigious *New England Journal of Medicine*, "Since the battle against cardiovascular disease was joined in mid-century, the news from the cardiovascular front has been almost uniformly positive. . . . An almost unbroken series of positive developments has encouraged the perception that the war against cardiovascular disease has been won or is well on its way to being won."[11]

In a 1996 editorial in *Science* magazine, Professors Michael S. Brown and Joseph L. Goldstein, winners of the Nobel Prize in Medicine in 1985, argue that progress against heart attacks will continue: "Heart attacks were recognized as a public health problem only in this century. They are likely to lose this notoriety in the next. The reason? Four decades of progress in understanding cholesterol and the lipoproteins that carry it in blood plasma."[12] Reviewing evidence from a variety of studies of animals, human populations, and clinical experiences, Brown and Goldstein suggest that even in the presence of other risk factors, lowering cholesterol with lifestyle changes and new drugs can do much to reduce heart disease.

The major goal now is to develop a noninvasive screening method to detect coronary artery disease in its early stages. Then, "exploitation of recent breakthroughs . . . may well end coronary heart disease as a major public health problem early in the next century."[13] Others second these optimistic predictions. Two other leading medical researchers state that "[t]he past decade has seen remarkable progress in clinical and basic research and many areas of opportunity are promising. The pace of current progress in clinical and basic research is such that remarkable improvement in the quality and length of life for those at risk for cardiovascular disease is likely."[14] Future advances involving a variety of new diagnostic techniques, medications, treatment procedures, and understandings of the sources of heart disease will no doubt help maintain the positive momentum. These advances may even make it possible to predict and treat the disease long before it occurs.[15]

We often hear the opposite: poor diet and limitations of modern medicine threaten our health and well-being. Although room for improvement always remains, the facts concerning heart disease demonstrate enormous progress rather than failure.

## CONTINUING CHALLENGES

Success in dealing with heart disease has in some ways resulted in a sense of complacency.[16] Less common, but more intractable diseases of cancer and AIDS have grabbed the most attention and garnered the most research funding in recent years. Despite progress, however, heart disease remains a crucial public health problem that requires continued vigilance. Jan I. Breslow, a former president of the American Heart Association, notes that lack of funding for cardiovascular research can slow progress toward the goal of eliminating heart disease as a major public health problem.[17]

Challenges certainly remain in the battle against heart disease. With the aging of the population, the numbers of persons with heart disease at older ages will increase despite progress in preventing and treating the problem among the young and middle-aged. Even at younger ages, blacks and females have not enjoyed the same decline in heart disease as white males. Those with low socioeconomic status and in southern regions of the country continue to have particularly high rates of heart disease. Worldwide, the growth of heart disease in developing nations can counter improvements in more developed nations. Surprisingly, coronary heart disease is expected to become the leading cause of death among residents of developing nations by 2020 and contribute substantially to the world-wide burden of disease.[18]

Some worry that trends toward healthier lifestyles may not continue. Although the typical diet today contains less fat than decades ago, the downward trend appears to have stalled. Diabetes and obesity are rising, and improvements made in reducing hypertension in recent decades appear to have ended. Declining rates of smoking have also slowed, particularly among young men and women. These changes may have already slowed the decline in heart disease and suggest that room for continued improvement remains.[19]

Recognizing new challenges in dealing with heart disease, however, does not negate what has been accomplished. The progress has been substantial. Along with lower death rates from heart disease, the past several decades have brought increased knowledge about the causes and treatment of the disease. Some background on how the heart works and what happens when it does not work can help to understand the growth of this knowledge.

## HOW THE HEART WORKS

The heart is a pump with four chambers that work in amazing harmony. First, blood filled with carbon dioxide and waste products of cell metabolism returns from the body in veins to the upper-right chamber (or right atrium) of the heart. Second, the blood enters through a valve into the lower-right chamber (or right ventricle). From the right ventricle, the blood is pumped under low pressure through the pulmonary artery to the lungs, where it releases the carbon dioxide and absorbs oxygen. Third, the oxygenated blood returns through the pulmonary vein to the heart in the upper-left chamber (or left atrium). Fourth, the blood then enters through a valve into the lower-left chamber (or left ventricle). From the left ventricle, the blood is pumped under high pressure through the aorta into arteries that will carry it throughout the body. During this process, heart valves control the movement of blood across the chambers. Much like one-way doors, they let blood into a chamber but not back out.

The process repeats on average 72 times a minute, over 100,000 times a day, over 37 million times a year, and nearly 3 billion times in a life. It pumps around 4,000 gallons of blood a day. For a muscle that is only a bit larger than the size of one's fist and weighs only 10 to 20 ounces, or about the same as a can of soda, the heart shows exceptional strength and endurance. The left side of the heart is particularly thick and strong because it has to contract enough to send the blood throughout the body (rather than to the nearby lungs).

Unlike other muscles, the heart never rests and proves essential to the functioning of all parts of the body. Like the rest of the body, the heart needs oxygenated blood. Since it cannot absorb blood directly through its walls, it depends on three important coronary arteries to nourish the muscle (*coronary* comes from a Greek word meaning "like a crown" and reflects the fact the coronary arteries fit over the heart like a crown). In fact, 10 percent of the blood pumped by the heart goes through these arteries.

To start the pumping action, the heart generates electrical signals from its own bioelectrical system rather than receiving impulses from the brain. The signals trigger the heart muscle to contract, but the contractions must be synchronized among the four chambers to make the pumping of the heart efficient. We speak of a heartbeat, but the heart contraction actually involves two closely spaced movements stimulated by the electrical system. The two upper chambers contract first, and then the two lower chambers follow an instant later. We refer to the heart as systolic when it is contracted and pumping blood out and diastolic when it is relaxed and filling with blood. These terms correspond to the components of blood pressure, or the force exerted against the arteries, with systolic the upper number and diastolic the lower number.

## MISCONCEPTIONS ABOUT THE HEART

Knowledge about how the heart works has emerged slowly throughout human history, and misunderstandings have lasted for thousands of years.

Primitive peoples had a good sense of the importance of the heart and blood: the beat of the heart matched the pulse of blood vessels, death ended the flow of blood, and a wound to the heart area—the center of the body—produced much blood. However, they had little understanding of the structure and function of the heart and circulation. The first systematic study of the heart came from the Greeks about 400 B.C. An unknown author described the two great vessels leading to the heart and the valves between the vessels and the heart chambers but identified only two rather than four chambers.[20] Not for another 130 years, in 270 B.C., was it discovered that the heart works as a pump and contains four chambers. A physician in Alexandria, Egypt, correctly concluded that blood enters the heart through the veins, and that the veins and arteries were connected, but he believed that air, rather than blood, flowed through the arteries.

A major—yet still incomplete—advance in the understanding of the workings of the heart came from the greatest of Greek physicians, Galen (A.D. 129–ca. 199). Galen recognized that the heart pumped blood rather than air through the arteries, saw the importance of the heart valves in preventing the blood from flowing backwards, and made several other important discoveries. Although human dissection was outlawed, Galen discovered much from experiments on live farm animals. After learning how to cut animals open without killing them, he could observe a beating heart.[21] Based on his experiments and the four hundred books he wrote on physiology, Galen's fame spread, and scholars and physicians accepted his word without question for the next 1,300 years.

However, Galen made mistakes that others continued to repeat. For example, he thought that invisible openings existed between the right and left sides of the heart that allowed blood to pass directly across chambers (when, in fact, blood goes to the lungs from the right side and returns from the lungs to the left side). He also thought that air and blood flowed separately to the heart chamber where they mixed. The errors of Galen and other physicians at the time likely resulted from their study of animal hearts, which differ in important ways from human hearts. In addition, the hearts moved so quickly, and so much was hidden behind the heart walls and within the vessels, that it was easy to make mistakes.

Physicians in Italy in the sixteenth century made the first efforts to correct the long-standing misconceptions about how the heart works.[22] Despite facing intense criticism, even hatred, for challenging the long-accepted beliefs of the Greeks and Romans, brave scholars demonstrated that no opening existed between the left and right sides of the heart. They further realized that blood exited from the right side of the heart, filtered through the lungs, mixed with air, turned bright red in color, and returned to the left side of the heart. The right and left side of the heart thus beat simultaneously, although for different purposes—one to send blood to the lungs and one to send the blood recently returned from the lungs to the rest of the body. Much remained to be learned about the heart and circulation, but progress toward a modern understanding had begun.

## WHAT CAN GO WRONG

Heart disease is more than a single ailment but includes a variety of problems in the functioning of the many parts of the heart. Indeed, one major problem originates from disease of the blood vessels that feed the heart rather than from the heart itself. Much can go wrong with the operation of the heart and its blood vessels. Corresponding to the structure of the heart, the problems can be divided into several groups.

### Coronary Heart Disease

The primary cause of heart disease and death from heart disease in modern societies is the inability of the coronary arteries to deliver the blood and oxygen needed by the heart muscle. Since the heart requires a continuous supply of blood, any blockage of the coronary arteries threatens the ability of the heart to operate. The most common cause of coronary heart or artery disease is atherosclerosis—a progressive development of material that becomes attached to the walls of the coronary arteries and restricts the flow of blood. The material or "plaque" consists of cholesterol deposits, calcium, and abnormal cells, and its buildup reflects blood vessel disease more generally.

Plaque serves to progressively narrow the artery and makes it difficult for blood to flow through to the heart muscle. The coronary arteries also become less flexible when filled with plaque (*sclerosis* means hardness) and help less in propelling the blood through the vessel. More seriously, even if a small plaque ruptures, it can trigger clotting of the blood within the artery that seriously obstructs the blood flow. This is the major cause of a coronary "event" or "acute coronary syndrome."

Individuals may experience symptoms from not getting enough blood through the coronary arteries. The lack of blood and oxygen to the heart muscle creates a pressure-like warning pain in or around the chest, shoulders, neck, or arms termed *angina pectoris.* The connection of the nerves around the heart to other parts of the body results in a diffuse pain. The symptoms usually subside with rest or medication but nonetheless indicate that the muscle is lacking oxygen. In other cases, the lack of oxygen to the heart muscle does not cause clear warning signals of pain. Ischemia or the lack of oxygen to the heart muscle can be all the more serious when it involves no angina or warning pain.

A myocardial infarction or heart attack occurs when a coronary artery becomes completely blocked, and the heart muscle supplied by that artery dies. *Myocardial* comes from *myocardium*, the technical term for the heart (in Greek, *myo* means muscle, and *kardia* means heart); the term *infarction* means death of the muscle cells. The seriousness of the heart attack depends on the amount of the heart muscle that dies. A myocardial infarction usually stems from the sudden rupture of an atherosclerotic plaque and subsequent clotting and blocking of the artery. The victim feels a squeezing pain in the chest that spreads to other parts of the upper body and is accompanied by sweating, nausea, or fainting; the pain may also simulate severe indigestion or heartburn. Not all chest pain results from a heart attack—similar feelings can come from indigestion, anxiety, or benign heart conditions. However, if the pain and symptoms are severe or last for more than 15 minutes, they probably require immediate medical attention.

### Cardiac Arrhythmia

Irregular heartbeats, or cardiac arrhythmia, can be too slow or too fast. When the heart rhythm is too slow (bradycardia), the part of the heart that generates electrical impulses becomes damaged, and the impulses may become weak or insufficient. Another form of bradycardia involves a condition called heart block, which prevents the electrical impulses from reaching the two lower chambers of the heart or the ventricles. When the heart rhythm is too fast (tachycardia), the disorderly contraction can limit the ability of the heart to pump blood to the body. Most seriously, ventricular fibrillation involves chaotic electrical impulses and the independent contraction of muscle fibers that halt meaningful contraction of the ventricles. This results in the stoppage of blood flow to the body, the loss of consciousness in a few seconds, and, without intervention, death in a few minutes.

Other types of arrhythmia include premature ventricular contractions that produce an "extra heartbeat" in the lower chambers. Premature ventricular contractions are generally benign unless they reflect other underlying heart problems. Atrial fibrillation (also known as flutter) occurs when the upper chambers beat irregularly and rapidly. Although not as serious a problem as ventricular fibrillation, atrial fibrillation causes the upper and lower chambers to beat irregularly, leads to clotting inside the heart and can result in a stroke if a clot breaks off and travels to the brain.

### Valvular Heart Disease

There are several causes of valvular heart disease, or the inadequate operation of the heart valves, such as rheumatic fever, congenital heart disease, cardiac dilation, and age-related calcification of the valves. However, the condition usually shows in one of two ways. First, the valve openings become too narrow and make it difficult for the blood to move from one chamber to the next. This is called valvular stenosis and leads to increased pressure in the heart chamber behind the valve. Second, the valves become incompetent so that blood leaks back across the valves when they are supposed to be closed. This is called valvular regurgitation and causes the heart chambers to dilate with extra blood.

In more extreme cases, both types of valvular problems can lead to congestive heart failure. Unlike the death of heart tissue from a heart attack, heart failure refers to the improper pumping of the heart, and congestive refers to the resulting buildup of fluids in the body. For example, if valvular problems affect the right atrium of the heart, blood is not properly absorbed from the veins, and edema or swelling of the liver, abdomen, and legs can result. If valvular problems affect the left atrium, then fluids accumulate in the lungs and make breathing difficult.

## Cardiomyopathy

Cardiomyopathy refers to diseases of the heart muscle. If the muscle of the left ventricle becomes weak, the amount of blood pumped in each heart beat drops, and the body does not receive its full quotient of blood. Called dilated cardiomyopathy, this problem results in shortness of breath, weakness, fatigue, and leg swelling and can produce life-threatening arrhythmia.

Hypertension or high blood pressure weakens the heart by making the vessels less elastic and the muscle walls thick and stiff. The inelasticity then requires the heart to pump harder to send the blood through the body. With the increased strain, the heart can become enlarged, and the enlargement can produce heart failure. Hypertrophic cardiomyopathy involves an inherited tendency of the ventricular muscle to thicken. This weakens the efficiency of the heart pumping and can cause sudden death in young athletes.

## Heart Failure

Heart failure is not a specific disease. Rather, it describes a group of symptoms involving the inability of the heart to pump enough blood to meet the body's needs. Heart failure results from several underlying problems, including valve problems, cardiomyopathy, high blood pressure, and damaged heart tissue from a heart attack. These underlying problems weaken the heart enough that the blood does not properly circulate. Consequently, the body tissue does not get the nutrients and oxygen it needs and does not get its waste materials removed. Shortness of breath and fatigue result, as does the accumulation of fluids in the lungs, feet, legs, and trunk. Because heart failure often involves the congestion of the tissues and lungs with fluid, it is often called congestive heart failure.[23]

## WILLIAM HARVEY: THE HEART AND BLOOD CIRCULATION

In 1628, William Harvey published *An Anatomical Treatise on the Motion of the Heart and Blood in Animals*. Historians of medicine consider it one of the most important books ever published on physiology, one similar in significance to Newton's work nearly 50 years later on gravity and the movement of the planets for modern physics. A serious and studious young man, Harvey went to study medicine in Italy, where he observed his professors dissecting human corpses. He returned to England to obtain a doctorate in medicine from Cambridge University, joined the teaching staff at St. Bartholomew's Hospital at London, and lectured at the Royal College of Physicians. He later served as the royal physician for King James I and King Charles I of England.

Harvey was the first to recognize that blood circulates through the body as a result of the pumping action of the heart. Although such an assertion seems obvious now, it represented a major change in the understanding of the time. Since Galen, physicians had thought that the body continuously created blood from food and "consumed" the blood as it moved to muscles and organs. By measuring the amount of blood pumped by the heart, Harvey revealed the fallacy of this assertion. His calculations demonstrated that the blood pumped by the heart in 30 minutes far exceeded the weight of the body. This much blood could not possibly be created anew but must instead recirculate through the body, each time transferring nutrients rather than being used directly. Harvey further demonstrated that blood moves away from the heart in the arteries to the veins and returns to the heart through the veins. Without a microscope, he could not see the tiny capillaries that connect the arteries to the veins, but his reasoning correctly led to the inference that such connections must exist.

In straightforward and logical wording, Harvey revolutionized thinking about the heart and circulation of the blood: "It is absolutely necessary to conclude that the blood in the animal body is impelled in a circle, and is in a state of ceaseless movement; that this is the act or function which the heart performs by means of its pulse, and that it is the sole and only end of the movement and contradiction of the heart."[24] Although his claims proved accurate, the criticism of his work by those unwilling to accept new truths damaged Harvey's reputation. He suspected as much would happen: "But what remains to be said upon the quantity and source of blood which thus passes, is of so novel and unheard of character, that I not only fear injury to myself from the envy of a few, but tremble lest I have mankind at large for my enemies."[25] Despite such criticism, history soon proved Harvey's work to be correct, and his insights created a basis on which medical science and cardiology could build.

## CORONARY ATHEROSCLEROSIS

Coronary artery or heart disease is by far the major cause of death in the United States—comprising about 63 percent of all heart disease deaths in 1998. Since it results from the buildup of plaque in the coronary arteries, it is a blood vessel disease as well as a form of heart disease. Coronary heart disease is not an event but a condition that progresses from mild to severe. The progression is complex and not fully understood, but it involves multiple factors.

### Cholesterol

Cholesterol is a fatty substance that the body uses to help form cell membranes and manufacture vitamin D and certain hormones such as estrogen. We ingest cholesterol in our food, but in the absence of such food, the liver can manufacture all the cholesterol the body needs. Cholesterol is one type of blood lipid (triglycerides are another). More important than cholesterol alone are lipoproteins that combine protein and lipids and transport cholesterol to cells. Low-density lipoproteins (LDL) enclose and transport cholesterol to cells and can accumulate in artery walls. Called the bad cholesterol, LDL contributes to heart disease. High-density lipoprotein (HDL) carries cholesterol back to the liver for processing and disposal and may even remove cholesterol from the artery walls. In contrast to bad cholesterol, this good cholesterol protects against heart disease. Common blood lipid tests now compare the level of total cholesterol (low- and high-density lipoproteins) to the level of high-density lipoproteins.

Evidence that elevated levels of cholesterol increase the risk of a heart attack by contributing to the buildup of plaque along the walls of the coronary arteries comes from three sources.[26] First, animals with low levels of LDL have no atherosclerosis, and raising LDL in animals universally causes the disease. Second, human populations with low LDL have little atherosclerosis, and the disease increases in proportion to LDL in all populations studied. Third, trials of drugs called statins that lower LDL also reduce heart attacks. However, elevated cholesterol represents just one of numerous risk factors. Many people with high LDL cholesterol (or high ratios of total cholesterol to HDL) do not have heart attacks, and many who have heart attacks do not have high cholesterol.

### Blood Clots

When a blood clot (or thrombus) lodges in a major artery (called atherothrombosis), it can become part of the plaque and narrow the artery. Blood clots protect and repair an injured part of a blood vessel but at the same time can grow so large as to block the flow of blood. Ideally, anti-clotting elements in the blood balance clotting elements, but under some circumstances, the clot does not get dissolved and accumulates LDL cholesterol and immune cells that contribute to plaque buildup. Certain kinds of cholesterol may reduce the ability of the body to naturally dissolve blood clots in blood vessels. In addition, high levels of a molecule called fibrinogen that forms the strands of the blood clot can exacerbate clotting problems.

### Insulin

The pancreas releases insulin into the bloodstream to help bring sugar and fat to the body's cells, but elevated levels can lead to a faster heart rate and to high blood pressure. High sugar levels and high insulin can also damage the lining of the arteries and raise LDL cholesterol.

### The Immune System

When immune cells called macrophages take residence just inside the artery wall, they can attract LDL cholesterol—particularly the damaged or oxidized LDL cholesterol. The uptake of cholesterol can then transform the immune cells into foam cells, which in turn accumulate into fatty streaks and contribute to the buildup of plaque. In addition, the immune cells release a substance that can inflame the artery wall, much as an allergic substance might inflame the sinus lining. This inflammation also promotes the development of fatty streaks and plaque buildup. Children as young as age 10 have fatty streaks in their arteries that may later develop into artery-clogging plaques, which highlights the fact that the development of atherosclerosis is a lifelong process rather than a sudden event.

### Lipoprotein(a)

Beginning in the 1990s, a possible explanation of heart disease based on the action of a particle in the blood called lipoprotein(a) emerged.[27] The particle helps repair torn blood vessels but may have the side effect of promoting blood clots in the coronary arteries. It does so by inhibiting the effectiveness of a similar protein that dissolves blood clots. When in excess, lipoprotein(a) thus promotes atherosclerosis. Since the level of lipoprotein(a) in the blood correlates with heart disease, varies greatly across individuals, and is stable over time, it may serve as a useful indicator of the risk of a heart attack.

## INJURIES TO THE ARTERY WALL

Elevated cholesterol, blood clotting, high insulin, and immune response all contribute to the buildup of plaque, but the process may begin with an injury to the artery wall. The initial injury may come from a disturbance of the blood flow, hypertension, infections, immune-system response, chemicals from tobacco smoke, high blood sugar, or a variety of minor events. Once the lining of the wall is injured, the cells become inflamed, macrophages attract lipids and form foam cells, and platelets begin to adhere to the wall to heal the wound. The end result is atherosclerosis—a blood vessel disease that blocks flow of blood to the heart.

In this sense, atherosclerosis is an inflammatory disease that does not result simply from high lipid or fat particles in the blood. Chronic inflammation of the artery wall from injury leads to repair efforts involving immune cell response, cholesterol absorption, and blood clotting, which can produce atherosclerosis, instability of plaque, potential heart attacks, and strokes. Indeed, the emergence of atherosclerosis differs little from other chronic inflammatory diseases. Much as inflammation in the liver leads to cirrhosis or inflammation in the joints leads to rheumatoid arthritis, inflammation in the artery wall leads to atherosclerosis.[28] In fact, a marker of inflammation called the C-reactive protein appears to predict risk of heart disease and can be measured in a screening test.

By promoting injury and inflammation of the artery wall, infections may play a crucial role in promoting heart disease—one more important than once thought. Researchers have discovered associations between coronary heart disease and the presence of certain persistent bacterial and viral infections such as helicobacter pylori, chlamydia pneumonia, and cytomegalovirus. For example, tests have found antibodies for chlamydia pneumonia in surprisingly large parts of the population and in even higher proportions of heart attack patients (around 70 percent).[29] Once infecting a person, the bacteria can rupture or inflame the artery wall in ways that promote the development of blockages. Other infectious agents, not currently known as associated with heart disease, may also have harmful effects.[30]

The potential importance of infections offers a new perspective on heart disease, one that highlights continuity with the diseases of the past. As infection by external bacteria and viruses once killed people quickly, they now may kill people slowly by producing the injury and inflation of the arteries that promote atherosclerosis and heart disease. The connection between infections and heart disease is less clear than the connection between, say, smallpox or scarlet fever and death, but it may well exist anyway.

Many diseases of the past, such as tuberculosis and peptic ulcers, were once viewed as lifestyle diseases but turned out to be caused by infections. If similar processes occur for heart disease, then attributing the problem to lifestyles alone may be a serious mistake. Lifestyles certainly relate to heart disease, just as they relate to tuberculosis and ulcers, but lifestyles alone may not identify the original or underlying cause of the disease.

If infections that injure the artery wall are central to the development of heart disease, it bodes well for future treatment. As we have had much success in the past in dealing effectively with infectious diseases, we may be able to identify those infected with chlamydia pneumonia or helicobacter bacterium and treat them with antibiotics well before the infections come to produce serious heart disease. Such treatments would be easier than efforts to change the diet, exercise, smoking habits, and blood pressure of large parts of the population. Indeed, the use of newly discovered antibiotics in the 1940s and 1950s may have had the unintended but beneficial side effect of contributing to falling heart disease in the 1960s and 1970s.

However, studies thus far have not conclusively demonstrated the importance of these infections.[31] Although certain bacteria are found in arterial plaque of victims of heart disease, it is difficult to prove that the bacteria cause the disease—perhaps existing plaque attracts rather than results from infectious organisms. The issue is currently the subject of intense international research activity, but studies face a problem: the antibodies of chlamydia pneumonia are hard to measure, and the bacteria are hard to culture. That makes it difficult to diagnose and treat the infection, and research on the effects of the infections on heart disease reveals mixed results.[32]

If continued research demonstrates the importance of infections, it might help solve a puzzle that confronts heart researchers and practitioners. Fully half of all patients with coronary heart disease do not have any of the six established risk factors: hypertension, high cholesterol, cigarette smoking, diabetes mellitus, marked obesity, and physical inactivity.[33] Such risk factors also fail to explain fully differences across populations and changes over time in the degree of coronary heart disease. For example, a study of trends in 21 countries from the mid-1980s to the mid-1990s showed that major risk factors explained only 15 percent of the changes in coronary events among men and 40 percent of the changes among women.[34] Others claim that established risk factors actually explain 75 percent of the incidence of coronary heart disease.[35] In any case, a good portion of heart disease mortality remains unexplained, which further emphasizes the need for continued efforts to understand the underlying causes.

---

## YOUNG PEOPLE AND HEART DISEASE

Anthony Bates, a 6-foot, 280-pound junior defensive tackle on the football team and an honors student at Kansas State University, was found slumped unconscious over the steering wheel of the pickup truck he was driving. The cause of death? Enlargement of the heart, or hypertrophic cardiomyopathy. Bates was one of hundreds of otherwise healthy young athletes who have died from this malady. Basketball stars Hank Gaithers of Marymount University and Reggie Lewis of the Boston Celtics were others. Many lesser-known high school and college athletes have also died from hypertrophic cardiomyopathy despite their young age and apparent top physical shape.[36]

Although heart problems usually occur in middle and old age, these prominent examples indicate that the risks affect youth as well. The numbers of young people who die of heart disease may be small, but the early loss of life makes youthful heart disease all the more serious.

Congenital and acquired are the two types of heart disease in children. Congenital heart disease is the result of defects present at birth; acquired heart disease develops during childhood and youth. Approximately 40,000 babies are born each year with congenital heart defects (about 8 out of every 1,000 infants born).[37] More than 1 million Americans alive today were born with heart defects. Heart defects claim the lives each year of close to 4,300 young people, but many others survive after surgery to correct the problem. Approximately 150,000 surgical procedures were performed on children age 15 or younger in 2000.

Children are also susceptible to behavioral and environmental factors that affect their risk of developing heart disease as they age. Like hypertrophic cardiomyopathy, coronary artery disease often begins in the teens and progresses from there as a person grows older. Coronary artery disease is found in boys and girls as young as 15 years old. Fatty streaks in the arteries can form by the teenage years, and hard plaques can form by young adulthood. Complicating the risk of coronary artery disease is the presence of additional risk factors. A 2001 survey of students in grades 9 through 12 found that 38.5 percent of males and 29.5 percent of females said they currently used tobacco. Most people who use tobacco begin before they turn 18, and the most common age at which people begin to smoke is 14 or 15 years. Many children are obese, do not get enough exercise, or have high cholesterol, which, like smoking, affects their likelihood of eventually developing heart disease.[38]

Approximately 4,000 children, youth, and young adults die each year of a disease known as long QT syndrome or sudden arrhythmia death syndrome (SADS). People with the disease, in many cases otherwise healthy, can experience sudden loss of consciousness and sudden cardiac death. Symptoms often first appear in the preteen or teenage years but can begin any time from infancy to middle age. Usually inherited, the syndrome affects the heart's electrical functioning and predisposes a person to an accelerated heart arrhythmia. Long QT syndrome is considered treatable, and patients showing signs of the disease, such as unexplained fainting after exercise, emotional distress, or being startled, can be diagnosed and treated if identified early. Some European countries have developed national programs to identify the problem in school children that could be usefully implemented in the United States.

## SOURCES OF PROGRESS AGAINST HEART DISEASE

Although many questions remain about the causes of coronary artery and other heart disease, researchers have attempted to document in general terms the major sources of the improvements in mortality rates. These sources are several. Primary prevention reduces the incidence of heart disease in the general population through improved lifestyles. Secondary prevention reduces the risk of continued problems among heart patients through improved lifestyles. Secondary prevention also reduces the risk of continued problems among heart patients through medical and surgical treatments. Finally, diagnostic efforts can reduce the risk of heart disease by identifying persons who need to change their lifestyle or receive treatment early rather than late.

Overlap makes it difficult to identify precisely the contribution of each source to the downward trend in heart disease mortality. We nonetheless have a good sense of general trends. In brief summary, early declines in heart disease mortality during the 1970s stemmed largely from changes in lifestyles, but treatment of heart patients contributed secondarily to improved outcomes. In contrast, changes during the 1980s stemmed largely from improvements in treatment, but prevention also played a role. New research needs to identify the role of the varied forces in the 1990s, but it seems likely that trends in the 1980s will continue.

The chapters to follow explore the components and causes of the progress we have made against heart and blood vessel disease. Chapters 2–5 examine the contributions to progress against heart disease of medical changes involving emergency lifesaving techniques, early diagnostic methods, less-invasive medical treatments, and surgical procedures. Chapters 6–9 then examine the contribution to reducing heart disease of lifestyle changes involving tobacco use, diet, exercise, weight, and stress. Because researchers have found that coronary artery disease often follows a different course in women than it does in men,[39] chapter 9 discusses how heart disease trends and the sources of the trends differ by sex. After the review of medical and behavioral factors, chapters 10 and 11 offer an overview of the trends in heart disease over the past century and the likely advances to be made in the current century.

Even avoiding hyperbole, these changes represent a remarkable story of scientific discovery and social change. Only a few decades ago, scientists thought that we had come close to the maximum human life expectancy and that declining mortality rates over the twentieth century would slow and end. That the opposite has occurred—trends toward longer life have continued unabated into the twenty-first century—reflects the importance of progress against heart disease. Americans today enjoy a healthier and longer life than ever before. The chapters to follow explore these changes and the stories behind them.

# PART II

## Medicine

# CHAPTER 2

# Emergency Lifesaving Treatment

John Colven, a 62-year-old smoker with some history of heart problems, laid down in the bedroom of the home he shared with his wife in a suburb of Seattle, Washington, around noon because he didn't feel well.[1] At 12:50, his wife walked into the room to find him unconscious but gasping for air. Although she didn't know the technical details—his heart had gone into ventricular fibrillation and stopped pumping blood—she knew the situation was serious and immediately called 911. John's heart was in fact quivering uncontrollably rather than contracting and relaxing in a coordinated way. Unresponsive to the world around him and unable to get oxygen to his brain, he was already clinically dead and would be biologically or irretrievably dead in five minutes. That he survived clinical death with no apparent long-term harm demonstrates the progress made in emergency heart treatment.

In John's case, the 911 dispatcher immediately notified two nearby sets of emergency medical technicians (EMTs) and then by phone guided John's wife through cardiopulmonary resuscitation (CPR). Because two firefighters with EMT training were only one mile away, they arrived at the house at 12:54 to find the wife continuing to give CPR. Taking over, they immediately saw the seriousness of the situation. At 12:57, they gave John an electrical shock with a defibrillator to get the heart beating again. The effort failed, but a second shock was successful. The EMTs then inserted a tube down John's throat so he could breath oxygen from an attached bottle. However, the pulse remained weak, and John's heart stopped once more. Two more electric shocks brought the heart back, and the pulse became stronger. Paramedics arrived at 1:03 and connected an intravenous (IV) to administer drugs that would help keep the heart beating at a regular pace. Put on a stretcher and brought to the hospital emergency room, John continued to receive treatment until he could be safely moved to the coronary care unit and eventually to a regular hospital room. In a few weeks, he returned back to his home nearly fully recovered.

The journal *New Jersey Medicine* reported a similar story:

In April 1998, R.R., aged 72 (a man with no prior history of cardiac disease), was leaving his house with two friends to play golf when he suddenly collapsed. One friend initiated CPR, and the other called 911 on his cellular phone. A Chatham police squad arrived within three minutes; the police "first responder" applied a portable automated external defibrillator (AED) to the unresponsive patient. The AED instructed the first responder to push the shock button. Pulse and blood pressure were immediately restored, and the patient was brought to the Overlook Hospital Emergency Room. The patient subsequently awakened, had a cardiac catheterization revealing severe three-vessel coronary artery disease, and then underwent successful coronary bypass surgery. Two and a half years later he remained asymptomatic and was seen in the office of his cardiologists for a routine semiannual exam. Later that same day he was scheduled to play golf with the same two friends who had previously saved his life.[2]

Yet another instance of the restoration of life involved someone young and, by all appearances, healthy. Kayla Burt, a 20-year-old guard on the University of Washington women's basketball team, fell off her bed and fainted while watching television with several other teammates in her Seattle apartment. Her friends called 911, and the dispatcher guided them through CPR until paramedics arrived. "Burt was later found to have Long QT Syndrome, an electrical disorder that causes the heart to beat irregularly. 'I'm lucky as anyone has ever been lucky,' said Burt, who can no longer play but whose scholarship will be honored. 'My heart was stopped. I was dead.' "[3]

These stories illustrate the potential of emergency medical treatment to save the lives of people whose hearts have stopped pumping blood. Just 50 years ago, John Colven, R.R., Kayla Burt, and others like them would certainly not have survived; today, successful lifesaving efforts in such circumstances are routine. As Dr. Mickey S. Eisenberg, one of the nation's foremost authorities and advocates of cardiac resuscitation, puts it, "For the first time in the million-plus years of human existence, we have the ability to reverse death. It happens every day, in thousands of towns and cities around the world."[4] Not surprisingly, the development of CPR, defibrillators, coronary care units, 911 dispatchers, and EMTs occurred around the same time that the death rates from heart disease began to fall. Although precise numbers are hard to pinpoint, these developments likely contributed to the progress made against heart disease mortality.[5]

At the same time, the ability to resuscitate victims is limited—the vast majority of those who go through CPR, defibrillation, and emergency-room care die anyway. Contrary to many examples and to the dramatic portrayals of television and the movies, the more typical emergency life-saving efforts involve less-positive outcomes. Most often, a call to 911, use of CPR by a family member, defibrillator shocks by EMTs, and oxygen bottles and IVs by paramedics fail to revive the victim. With no indication of any success in returning the heart to its normal state, the paramedics still load the victims onto the stretcher and bring them to the hospital emergency room. Again, a team of doctors and nurses work diligently at revival before declaring the nonresponsive patients as dead. In the mean-time, family members, friends, and neighbors watch idly as the victims are taken by strangers in an ambulance and declared dead in the imper-sonal setting of a hospital.[6]

To what extent has emergency lifesaving medical treatment contributed to the decline in mortality from heart disease? If kept alive long enough, individuals with heart problems can later be treated with medications and lifestyle changes and in many cases can live a long and happy life. Emer-gency treatment could in this way have a long-term impact on life expec-tancy. However, much of the promise of emergency treatment has not yet been realized. Benefits certainly come to the individuals whose lives are saved by the treatment and to their families, but the relatively few suc-cesses may contribute only modestly to the mortality statistics. For others, the emergency treatment may destroy the dignity of the dying experience and remove control of the experience from relatives and friends to stran-gers. In addressing these issues, this chapter describes the emergency life-saving techniques that have emerged in recent decades and examines their contribution to progress against death from heart disease.

## TREATING SUDDEN CARDIAC ARREST

Cardiac arrest refers to the abrupt and immediate stoppage of the heart's ability to pump blood through the body. It differs from a heart attack, or myocardial infarction, in which the heart is deprived of oxygen but continues to beat. About 65 to 80 percent of the time, sudden cardiac arrest results from ventricular fibrillation—the chaotic and uncoordinated quivering of heart muscle fibers.[7] This condition prevents the pumping of blood throughout the body and results in respiratory arrest (the breathing is stopped) and sudden unconsciousness. Sudden cardiac arrest also re-sults from tachycardia (the excessively rapid beating of the heart) about 10 percent of the time, and from asystole (cardiac standstill) about 20 to 30 percent of the time.

Cardiac arrest largely results from three underlying heart disease con-ditions. First, it stems from myocardial infarction, or the death of heart tissue from a blockage of the coronary arteries. Second, it stems from ischemia or a lack of oxygen supplied to the heart muscle (but not the death of the tissue). And third, it stems from primary fibrillation due to an irregular heart rhythm, problems in the heart's electrical signals, and certain inherited heart problems such as hypertrophic cardiomyopathy and long QT syndrome. In rarer cases, sudden cardiac arrest can also result from recreational drug use.

If emergency intervention occurs early, cardiac arrest caused by ventricular fibrillation is highly treatable. The heart rhythm of the victim needs to be stabilized quickly, and the blood flow and breathing need to be restored. If resuscitated, about one-half of survivors of cardiac arrest live another four years or more. However, the longer the time between cardiac arrest and life support, the lower the chance of survival or the greater the chance of long-term harm among survivors. About 10 percent of the ability to restart the heart is lost with every minute the heart stays in fibrillation.[8] In hospitals, the success rate in restarting a heart undergoing ventricular fibrillation reaches 95 percent because of the ability to begin emergency treatment immediately; outside the hospital, the success rate is much lower because of the delay in giving treatment.

The potential importance of emergency treatment shows in a classic study of incidents of out-of-hospital cardiac arrest in Seattle, Washington. When CPR was initiated within 4 minutes and definitive therapy was delivered within 8 minutes, 43 percent of the victims survived ventricular fibrillation and were able to leave the hospital.[9] In contrast, only 7 percent survived to leave the hospital if CPR did not begin within 8 minutes, and no patients survived if untreated for 16 minutes.

Sadly, emergency treatment in most cases does not occur soon enough to be effective. "Only 2 to 5 percent of the 225,000 persons who have sudden cardiac arrest outside a hospital are successfully resuscitated. For those with ventricular fibrillation, these dismal statistics are in stark contrast to the high success rate when defibrillation is performed immediately after the onset of ventricular fibrillation."[10] The key to the success rate of emergency treatment for sudden cardiac arrest is delivering the immediate treatment that occurs in the hospital to those who experience the event outside the hospital.

In aiming to improve the odds of survival from sudden cardiac arrest, the American Heart Association has since the early 1990s presented treatment guidelines.[11] These guidelines emphasize the importance of a rapid sequence of intervention and the collaboration of the public and medical practitioners in guaranteeing quick treatment. As it involves four actions that are closely linked, the American Heart Association refers to the intervention as the "Chain of Survival." Each of the individual actions in the chain is necessary, but none is sufficient.

## ANCIENT RESUSCITATION STORIES

Reported attempts at resuscitation began with recorded history, and stories passed down from generation to generation likely preceded recorded history.[12] Ancient writings from Egypt dating back to 2000 B.C. mention restoring life through driving out evil spirits. In one Egyptian myth, the goddess Isis restores her husband by breathing into his mouth. Hebrew history preceding the Bible includes stories of midwives breathing life into newborn infants thought to be dead. The Talmud, a compilation of writings on Jewish civil and religious law that followed the Bible, also discusses the problem of breathing among newborns, recommending that "the new born is held so it should not fall on the earth and one blows into his nostrils."[13]

Perhaps most well known are instances of resuscitation in the Bible. In the first book of Kings in the Old Testament, the prophet Elijah lays himself on his landlady's dying son, whose illness was so severe that there was no breath left in him. Elijah first prayed and stretched himself along the sick child, "and the soul of the child came into him again, and he revived."[14] In the second book of Kings, the prophet Elisha is described using something closer to today's mouth-to-mouth resuscitation: "And when Elisha came into the house, behold the child was dead, and laid upon his bed. He went in therefore, and shut the door upon the twain, and prayed unto the Lord. And he went up and lay upon the child, and put his mouth upon his mouth, and his eyes upon his eyes, and his hands upon his hands; and he stretched himself upon him; and the flesh of child waxed warm. Then he returned, and walked in the house once to and fro; and went up, and stretched himself upon him; and the child sneezed seven times, and the child open his eyes."[15] Resuscitation as a modern medical technique emerged only recently, but the idea behind it has existed nearly as long as humankind.

## CHAIN OF SURVIVAL

### Early Access

The first link in the chain of survival, early access, requires immediate recognition of the symptoms of cardiac arrest and notification of the emergency medical system. The need to call 911 upon the sudden collapse and unconsciousness of a victim of cardiac arrest would seem obvious, but the effort is often slowed by uncertainty of bystanders about what happened, the difficulty of getting to a phone, confused statements to the dispatcher, and the time needed for the dispatcher to notify emergency personnel. Before calling the emergency number, persons may call friends or relatives for advice, wait for the victim to recover, slowly try to rouse the victim by shaking them gently or talking to them, or call a personal physician for help. All these actions slow the emergency intervention process. Educational programs of the American Heart Association and the Red Cross have done much, but can still do more, to teach the public about the signs of cardiac arrest and the appropriate action to take.

Establishment of and education about a 911 emergency phone number can help avoid the slow process of looking up phone numbers or mistakenly calling several phone numbers until finding the appropriate response. The successful implementation of the 911 number in the United States in the 1970s led to the creation of a common emergency number in the European community in the 1990s and therefore to the coverage of another 350 million people across the world by a standardized emergency system. Early access also relates to the ability of the ambulance to reach the victim promptly. However, beyond a certain threshold, adding more ambulances does little to improve the speed of arrival and is expensive and inefficient. Rather, greater public awareness and more efficient dispatching do the most to improve the speed of early access.

### Early CPR

The second link in the chain is early CPR. Since initiation of CPR by emergency personnel would in most cases occur too late to help the victim, basic CPR should be done by trained citizens at the same time as or immediately after notifying the emergency system. The goal of CPR is to produce enough blood flow to the brain to keep the patient viable until arrival of the EMTs, or in other words, to slow the dying process. By itself, CPR rarely can resuscitate a victim, but if delivered within four minutes of cardiac arrest, it can increase the likelihood of subsequent successful intervention. Those who receive CPR within four minutes are at least six times more likely to survive than those who receive CPR later.

Toward the goal of making early CPR widely available and training large parts of the population, the American Heart Association, the Red Cross, and numerous local organizations offer free courses on the technique that last only a few hours. As a result, more than 5 million Americans receive training each year and can contribute to this link in the chain of survival.[16] However, since the opportunity for most persons trained in CPR to use the technique in a real life-threatening situation occurs rarely, and often only many years after training, nonmedical personnel hesitate to use it. Moreover, when they do use it, they may make mistakes. Continued retraining can help deal with these problems, but in addition, the use of dispatcher-assisted CPR can help guide those with previous training through the procedure and even teach it to those who have had no CPR training. Dispatcher-assisted CPR (as used to help keep John Colven alive until help could arrive) also has the advantage of calming and directing the efforts of the emergency bystanders. The combination of training programs and dispatcher-assisted CPR in King County, Washington, increased the initiation of CPR by bystanders from 30 percent in 1980 to 60 percent in 1988.

CPR involves three steps, which are called the ABCs: airway, breathing, and circulation. First, the rescuer makes sure the victim's airways are clear by gently tilting the head back and opening the jaw. If removing obstructions from the mouth and moving the tongue out of the throat fails to clear the airway, it is necessary to perform the Heimlich maneuver to dislodge any blockage of the throat or voice box. Second, if breathing has stopped, artificial respiration or mouth-to-mouth ventilation should begin. With the airway open and the nose pinched closed, the rescuer exhales twice into the victim's mouth. Ideally, this will inflate the victim's lungs. Third, if no signs of blood circulation appear, the rescuer should externally compress the chest area. By kneeling next to the victim, placing the heel of one hand on the middle of the breastbone and placing the other hand on top of and interlocked with the first hand, the rescuer can press down about 1.5 to 2 inches and then release the pressure. At the rate of about 1 compression per second, the rescuer alternates 15 compressions with two breaths. Since this last step can place considerable physical demands on a single rescuer, CPR is more effectively performed by two people working in collaboration.

Although the instructions are straightforward, some risks come from use of the procedure. When performed on someone whose breathing and pulse have not stopped, CPR can cause (rather than relieve) cardiac arrest. Done incorrectly or too forcefully, CPR can damage internal organs. In addition, infants require special techniques. With these provisos, the technique is clearly helpful. According to the American Heart Association, the overall long-term survival rate for someone who has received CPR is about 16 percent. Although this figure may seem low, that percentage drops to just 6 percent when CPR is not administered.

The American Heart Association's latest CPR guidelines for laypeople have made some simplifications of past guidelines. Unlike previous recommendations, current recommendations do not require laypeople to check for a pulse before starting chest compression. Laypeople have difficulty reliably determining if a pulse is present, so it is best to look for other signs such as unconsciousness and lack of breathing movement. The current recommendations also suggest that chest compression should be used to attempt to remove obstructions from the throat before doing the Heimlich maneuver.

To simplify further the CPR procedure in ways that would make it possible for larger parts of the population to use it, recent experiments suggest that rescuers can begin with chest compression rather than assisted breathing.[17] The most important goal is to get blood that is already oxygenated to the body, and this is done through prompt, rapid, and forceful chest compression. Some studies of both animals and humans find that survival probabilities for traditional CPR and for chest compression alone do not differ significantly. Given that chest compression is easier and less distasteful than mouth-to-mouth resuscitation, bystanders may more willingly apply the former technique than the latter technique to strangers.

In one study of the alternative procedure in Seattle, for example, half the bystanders giving dispatcher-assisted CPR were instructed to use chest compression alone and half were instructed to use both assisted breathing and chest compression. The results demonstrate that the rate of survival to hospital discharge was greater among patients assigned to chest compression alone.[18] While recognizing the promise of this approach, the American Heart Association still recommends use of traditional CPR. The results for Seattle may not apply to other cities and areas, and chest compression alone can do little to help those with breathing problems rather than heart problems. More research may lead to changes in formal guidelines in the future.

### Early Defibrillation

Although CPR remains crucial to emergency treatment and can force blood to the brain through the body, it cannot restore the heart rhythm of the patient. Early defibrillation, the third link in the chain of survival, aims to do this. It involves delivering an electrical shock to the heart when the heartbeat is dangerously fast due to ventricular tachycardia or quivering due to ventricular fibrillation. Generally, the goal is to convert an ineffective cardiac rhythm into a normal, spontaneous rhythm. The notion that defibrillation can electrically shock a heart without electrical and muscle activity back into action is incorrect. A defibrillating shock reorganizes electrical activity rather than creates it, and such a shock offers virtually no chances of survival for victims without any electrical activity in the heart.

Like CPR, speed in intervention is essential for the effective use of a defibrillation shock. It should begin within at least five to six minutes of cardiac arrest. When done immediately, as in cases when cardiac arrest occurs under conditions supervised by medical personnel, defibrillation results in a survival rate of nearly 90 percent, but with each minute that passes, the chances for survival decrease by 10 percent. The American Heart Association aims to have those with cardiac arrest in the hospital treated by defibrillation within three minutes and those out of the hospital treated by defibrillation within five minutes.

Small and portable automatic external defibrillators (AEDs) allow laypersons as well as medical professionals to use them in lifesaving and can promote the goals of the American Heart Association. Once turned on and placed on the victim's chest, the AED reads the heart rhythm to determine if an electrical shock will be appropriate. In 80 percent of the cases, the instructions will be to give the shock, which requires only that the rescuer and bystanders not touch the patient to avoid the risk of accidental shock. In other cases, the AED reads not to shock when the procedure is not warranted. Implementation of an early defibrillation program in King County, Washington, raised survival rates of patients in ventricular fibrillation from 7 percent to 26 percent.

The American Heart Association estimates that 20,000 lives would be saved every year in the United States if the public had better access to AEDs. With this goal in mind, AEDs are being made available in airports, airplanes, stadiums, casinos, shopping malls, and golf courses, as well as in ambulances and fire rescue vehicles. Given public access to the machine, the use of a defibrillator has shifted from a medical procedure to a lay procedure. Since paramedics reach a victim on average about 12 minutes after collapse, the presence of an AED nearby and minimal training of laypeople would allow them to defibrillate victims rapidly.

The distribution of AEDs in busy public places has led to some encouraging results. American Airlines, for example, placed AEDs on all flights and trained all flight attendants in their use. "The program was highly effective for victims who were found to have ventricular fibrillation (13 of 13 of whom were successfully defibrillated and 40 percent of whom survived to discharge from the hospital with full neurological and functional recovery)."[19] In another study, the use of automated external defibrillators by trained security guards in gambling casinos improved the survival rate among patients experiencing cardiac arrest by 25 to 50 percent.[20]

The risks of error in use of the machines by laypeople appear small. Nonmedical personnel, even children, can learn to use the machines easily or follow the instructions of an emergency dispatcher. In a mock scenario, 15 11-year-old children took only 90 seconds to defibrillate a patient, compared with the 67 seconds taken by paramedics.[21] This result came with only a minute of verbal instruction and suggests that training for use of AEDs need not be extensive. Other studies show that AEDs are 90 percent effective (i.e., they correctly detect a rhythm that needs defibrillation) and 99 percent specific (i.e., they recommend not shocking when defibrillation is inappropriate).[22]

AEDs would be particularly valuable in the home, where 75 percent of cardiac arrests take place. The next step toward improving performance of the early defibrillation link may involve placement of AEDs in homes of high-risk individuals. At a cost of $3,000 per unit, AEDs are expensive for patients to purchase, but if produced in greater mass, the price of the machines may drop.[23] In any case, the evidence thus far of the use of AEDs by laypersons in the home has not been positive, but the potential to save the lives of those who collapse in private rather than in public places makes pursuit of this objective worthwhile.

### Advanced Cardiac Life Support

The last link involves more advanced procedures such as endotracheal intubation and IV medication that further improve the chances of survival. Intubation provides oxygen directly to the lungs but is difficult to perform, as the tube may not be properly inserted or may come loose. Other forms of oxygen delivery, such as the use of bag masks, can work effectively when intubation does not, but they also require special equipment and skills. Setting up an IV to deliver medications also requires special skills best left to paramedics or medical personnel. IVs may include medications such as lidocaine or amiodarone, which suppress irregularities in the heartbeat, and medications such as epinephrine and vasopressin, which constrict vessels, increase blood pressure, and improve circulation of the blood.

Paramedics, who receive one thousand to three thousand hours of classroom training and field instruction, perform such procedures in the United States (in many other nations, ambulances carry nurses and physicians). Although not as critical as defibrillation, intubation and intravenous medication delivered by paramedics can raise the probability of survival. A review of studies reveals that 16 percent of victims survive with the use of defibrillation alone. With the additional treatment by paramedics after defibrillation, survival goes up to 29 percent.[24] After treatment by paramedics, medical personnel in emergency rooms can continue these treatments and implement more advanced procedures. For example, anticlotting drugs, heart catheterization, and angioplasty can help deal with the coronary problems that often underlie cardiac arrest.

Finally, advanced life support extends to coronary care units (CCUs) in hospitals. In CCUs, heart monitors continuously send information to the nurses' station, which allows any renewed fibrillation to be recognized and treated immediately. Given the high probability of resuscitation if defibrillation occurs quickly, hospitals with CCUs have enjoyed a decline in case fatality rates. In addition, IV delivery of medications and liquid food, which does not require diverting blood to the digestive system, aids recovery of cardiac arrest patients in CCUs. Researchers note that the decline in coronary heart disease mortality in the mid-1960s occurred almost exactly at the same time as the implementation of CCUs.[25]

---

## LEONARD COBB AND THE SEATTLE MEDIC ONE PROGRAM

In 1969, Seattle, Washington, began one of the nation's first paramedic programs to deal with cardiac arrest outside the hospital. In the decades to follow, it became the nation's most successful program—one used as a model for other cities and parts of the country.[26] The efforts started with sending specially trained firefighters to treat victims of cardiac arrest at the scene, a practice now ordinary in most cities. They could perform CPR and give defibrillator shocks to restore the proper heart rhythm. While an important start, the use of emergency technicians alone could not properly treat many victims. Seattle added to the system by training more than 600,000 citizens in CPR during the last 30 years and by training emergency dispatch operators to give CPR instructions over the phone. The city also added paramedics, who would arrive on the scene after the firefighters to provide advanced life support. Several scientific studies have found high rates of resuscitation for victims of cardiac arrest in Seattle.

Seattle's success with resuscitation efforts comes in large part from the work of one physician, Dr. Leonard Cobb. As a professor of medicine at the University of Washington and director of cardiology at a Seattle hospital, Cobb read an article about the use of a mobile coronary care unit that sent physicians and nurses to the scene of suspected cardiac arrest in Belfast, Northern Ireland.[27] He didn't think that using physicians and nurses in Seattle would be a wise use of resources, but he contacted the Seattle fire chief about using firefighters to provide emergency heart treatment. With a grant, Cobb arranged to pay the salaries of 15 firefighters who would be trained in emergency heart-care procedures and to evaluate scientifically the success of the program. The program also purchased a large motor home that would serve as the first mobile care unit. It stayed at the hospital and would follow the firefighters to the scene to give more advanced heart care. Many of Cobb's colleagues opposed the effort. "Skeptics said this is potentially dangerous stuff—they'll be killing people left and right. It took strong-willed people to get the program going, people like Leonard Cobb."[28]

Cobb remembers a 17-year-old boy who was one of the first persons resuscitated in the Seattle program. "The boy was downtown in his father's office. After he went to the bathroom, somebody went in and found him slumped over unconscious. They called the unit and he had VF [ventricular fibrillation]. . . . [After a successful resuscitation], he was very slow to wake up; it took 10 days. He went back to finish high school and went skiing the following winter."[29] The program seemed successful in other ways. In its first year, the program resuscitated 61 patients, 31 of whom were successfully discharged from the hospital. In a segment on the program, the television show 60 Minutes called Seattle the best place in the country to have a heart attack. When a cut in funding from the grant threatened the program, Cobb led a fund-raising effort in the community that contributed $200,000 to the program.

In the 1970s, the program spread to the communities in King Country, Washington, that surround Seattle and now serves nearly 2 million people. The benefits of the program come at low cost. "In 1976 a series of county-wide levies was passed by voters to fund the program. The annual cost to the citizens is approximately 25 cents for every $1000 of assessed property valuation."[30] In Cobb's calculations, based on the experiences of the program during one year, it costs about $3,000 to save a life—$150,000 in 1970 to run a program that saved 50 lives that year.

## DEVELOPMENT OF EMERGENCY PROCEDURES

The progress made over the last several decades in emergency lifesaving techniques represents the accumulation of knowledge over several centuries. Although stories of resuscitation occur throughout history, the effort to develop sound scientific methods began in the late eighteenth century. Organized in 1774 in London, the Royal Humane Society aimed to develop and publicize ways to resuscitate victims of drowning and sudden heart attacks. The public showed much resistance to such efforts, viewing the revival of the dead as akin to witchcraft and magic. Indeed, some of the recommended methods today seem remarkably misdirected. Besides bleeding the victim from a vein, the Royal Humane Society at one time recommended blowing tobacco smoke with a bellows through the rectum and into the large intestines of the victims.[31] However, they later came to promote more sensible techniques such as rolling the body over a barrel, which would in a crude way compress the chest and help expel air from the lungs.

Modern CPR came in the late 1950s and early 1960s with the merging of the techniques of mouth-to-mouth resuscitation for artificial respiration and chest compression for artificial circulation. In 1958, Dr. Peter Safar showed that an airway obstructed by the tongue prevented effective mouth-to-mouth respiration, but that hyper-extending the neck with the head facing up would deal with this problem.[32] In 1962, researchers reported that external pressure on the chest wall could restore adequate circulation of the blood, provided that breathing was simultaneously restored by mouth-to-mouth ventilation.[33] Surgeons had known that if for some reason the heartbeat of a patient undergoing surgery stopped, they could revive the heart by massaging it by hand. This open-heart compression could, obviously, be used only in rare instances during ongoing surgery, but closed-chest or external compression could also circulate the blood.

Defibrillation in its modern form also emerged in the 1960s. The idea that an electrical machine could help resuscitate victims dates back to the Royal Humane Society, but scientific demonstrations of the potential use of electrical shocks began with Dr. Paul Zoll. First finding in the 1950s that he could stimulate the heart externally with electricity, Zoll and his colleagues in 1955 applied a single shock with electrodes across the chest of a 64-year-old woman undergoing ventricular fibrillation in the hospital. The shock stopped the fibrillation but did not restart the heart.[34] Over the next four months, Zoll had more success, but the machine giving the shock was large and heavy—not suitable for use outside the hospital.

In building on the efforts of Zoll and in further experimenting with defibrillation on animals, Dr. Bernard Lown found that direct current more consistently restored the proper rhythm of the heart than the alternating current of Zoll's machine.[35] In addition, the use of direct current made it possible for a battery to supply the electricity for the shock efficiently. This made the defibrillator portable and useful for treatment outside the hospital. Lown reported on his findings in 1962, which occurred at about the same time that CPR was emerging. Combined with the use of CPR to keep victims alive during the early minutes of cardiac arrest, the new defibrillation units could do much to improve survival rates.

A final key to the emergence of current emergency lifesaving techniques came from the use of mobile coronary care units. The success of CCUs in hospitals spawned the idea to put the intensive care equipment into a small truck or van. Such efforts began in Belfast, Northern Ireland, in 1966.[36] Physicians and nurses on call would travel with the mobile unit and provide much the same care at the scene to persons in cardiac arrest as they would to someone brought to the hospital. The idea spread to New York City, Charlottesville, Virginia, and Seattle, Washington. Physicians and nurses in the ambulances were replaced by paramedics and EMTs, who could provide initial support before bringing the patient into the hospital for more advanced care. The establishment of a universal 911 phone number in the 1970s made the use of ambulances all the more effective.

## EVALUATION OF THE EFFECTIVENESS OF EMERGENCY TREATMENT

In principle, early access, early CPR, early defibrillation, and advanced cardiac life support can effectively increase the survival odds of persons experiencing sudden cardiac arrest. In particular, those victims undergoing ventricular fibrillation and tachycardia—about 77 to 90 percent of all cases of cardiac arrest—have a high probability of revival.[37] Some reports find that for ventricular fibrillation, 40 percent of victims are resuscitated and hospitalized and 23 percent are discharged from the hospital, and that for tachycardia, 88 percent are resuscitated and hospitalized and 67 percent are discharged. The other 20 to 30 percent of the cases who experience other forms of cardiac arrest have virtually no chance of survival: only 9 percent are resuscitated and none are discharged from the hospital.[38]

Other reports suggest similarly high potential for successful resuscitation. If all four links in the chain of survival come together quickly, such as when CPR is started within four minutes of collapse and when advanced care (defibrillation, medications, endotracheal intubation) is instituted within eight minutes, there is a 43 percent probability of resuscitation, hospitalization, and discharge from the hospital.[39]

King County, Washington, has implemented all the links in the chain of survival and in many ways serves as a model of emergency lifesaving for other counties. In the county's largest city, Seattle, some 600,000 citizens have received CPR training, emergency dispatch operators can give CPR instruction over the phone, firefighters aim to arrive within three to four minutes and give defibrillator shocks, and paramedics aim to arrive within eight minutes to give advanced life-support care. From 1976 to 1987, the survival rate in King County fluctuated between 15 to 20 percent for all cardiac arrests and between 25 to 30 percent for ventricular fibrillation. This level of success may represent the practical limits for prehospital emergency care.

However, efforts to implement the system in many cities and counties have not reached the high success rate of King County. In New York City, the likelihood of being revived after cardiac arrest is only 1 percent, largely because slow traffic makes it difficult for emergency personnel to get to victims quickly.[40] In other cities with emergency lifesaving systems, revival rates vary from 7 to 18 percent. In rural areas where the emergency system is primitive and travel to distant places takes longer, lifesaving efforts fall to even lower levels. One estimate suggests that the national survival rate is "only 2 to 5 percent of the 225,000 persons who have sudden cardiac arrest outside a hospital."[41] In short, "The inherent time delays associated with delivery of EMS [Emergency Medical Services] and the resultant delays to onset of CPR and defibrillation, even when measured in minutes, preclude a significant impact on cardiac arrest mortality."[42]

Perhaps the failure to effectively implement all the links in many cities points to a need to make greater efforts to educate the public. The weakest link in the chain of survival comes from the lack of bystander-initiated CPR and the delay of defibrillation. These links might be strengthened by the use of chest compression alone and by encouraging the widespread access and use of AEDs.[43]

In any case, assuming a maximum success rate in practice of 20 to 30 percent, such as found in King County, allows some calculations of the effectiveness in saving lives. If the current survival rate equals 3 percent of the annual 400,000 cases of out-of-hospital cardiac arrest, then 12,000 people now survive. A 20 percent survival rate would yield an additional 68,000 lives saved. The American Heart Association suggests even more optimistically that implementing all lifesaving techniques throughout the United States could save between 100,000 and 200,000 people.[44]

These figures relate to changes over time in heart disease mortality. In examining the declining death rates from coronary heart disease from 1968 to 1976, one study calculated that about 5 percent of the observed decline resulted from prehospital resuscitation and care.[45] That is not a large percentage but nonetheless translates into thousands of lives saved. Assuming that improvement in techniques and the spread of emergency systems to new cities and areas has continued since 1976, the development of lifesaving techniques for those undergoing cardiac arrest may well have contributed in similar ways to more recent progress against heart disease. More improvement may yet come in the future if the goal of 20 percent survival is reached across the country.

Critics view these resuscitation goals as unreachable and the effort to resuscitate most victims as harmful.[46] Failed resuscitation, the most likely outcome of sudden cardiac arrest, reduces the quality and dignity of death by separating victims from loved ones and giving control of the dying experience to strangers. Moreover, the efforts to resuscitate may create false expectations among family members and friends, who, having seen television shows that exaggerate the success of CPR and defibrillation, believe the emergency procedures will have a high rate of success. In fact, since it largely fails, most merely watch their dying relative being taken away.

Regardless of the sometimes low success rate, advocates of emergency treatment view the procedures as life affirming.[47] Those successfully re-suscitated have a good quality of life, with two-thirds returning to their previous life with minimal impairment, one-quarter having moderate to severe impairment, and 5 percent requiring nursing care.[48] Although not appropriate for the frail elderly, chronically or terminally ill patients, and cases where lifesaving efforts involve trauma rather than a peaceful death, resuscitation remains the norm and likely will continue to be in the future.

# CHAPTER 3

# Diagnosing Heart Disease

On April 24, 1955, the most powerful man in the world, President Dwight D. Eisenhower, awoke in the early morning hours with severe chest pain. Although the story was kept secret at the time, a review of historical documents suggests doctors botched the diagnosis and put the president at considerable risk.[1] That he survived and successfully ran for a second term as president resulted as much from his determination and physical strengths as from his medical care. Several mistakes were made.

When called to deal with the president's chest pain, Eisenhower's personal physician, Dr. Howard M. Snyder, gave his patient morphine to reduce the pain and sat by the bedside. He made no effort to determine if the president had experienced a heart attack or to get immediate treatment for it. This wait-and-see response could easily have led to Eisenhower's death. Only when chest pain recurred 12 hours later did Dr. Snyder call for help and obtain an electrocardiogram of the electrical activity of Eisenhower's heart. It turned out that the president was indeed having a heart attack.

Mistakes and confusion followed. The chief cardiologist at Walter Reed Army Hospital concluded—as it turns out, wrongly—that Eisenhower had an even earlier undiagnosed heart attack, experienced a ventricular aneurysm as a result of the heart attack, and faced a grim prognosis. Dr. Paul Dudley White, a leading cardiologist from Boston, was then called in for consultation. He disputed claims of a previous heart attack and aneurysm and believed the recent heart attack was not as severe as others claimed. At a time when most doctors prescribed complete bed rest as the major treatment for heart disease, White advocated allowing patients to

resume normal activities and hoped Eisenhower would serve as a model
for the new recommendations.

Rejecting the advice of many of his doctors and family members, Eisenhower decided to run again for the presidency in 1956 and won the
election. His heart attack brought great publicity about the seriousness of
the disease to Americans but also exposed the inadequate means of diagnosing the problem. The delay and difficulties in making a diagnosis
threatened Eisenhower's life and illustrated the limited means physicians
had at the time to understand the seriousness and sources of heart disease
and heart attacks. Today, electrocardiograms and blood tests can quickly
determine if a person is experiencing or has had a heart attack. The availability of such tests in Eisenhower's time, along with further tests to diagnose the exact nature of the heart problem, would have led to
immediate attention and better treatment.

In the past, doctors specializing in internal medicine found cardiology
a difficult subspecialty because they had to base their diagnoses on listening to the heart and measuring its electrical activity.[2] While helpful and
still used today, these procedures often (as in the case for President Eisenhower) do not provide a clear indication of the source and degree of the
problem. Today, the development of advanced diagnostic procedures such
as nuclear imaging and catheterization has made diagnosis of heart disease easier and more accurate. By precisely identifying heart problems
and thereby allowing for appropriate treatment, the procedures have contributed importantly to the progress against premature mortality from
heart disease and improved the quality of life for millions.

This chapter reviews the diagnostic procedures used today to determine
the precise source of a patient's heart disease and suggests the most appropriate form of treatment.[3] Although researchers lack precise estimates
of the contribution of earlier and better diagnosis to the lessening of heart
disease mortality, evidence suggests that the diagnostic improvements
have helped considerably.

## COMMON METHODS OF DIAGNOSIS

### Health History and Physical Exam

A health history and physical exam, done routinely for people of all
ages, represents a preliminary but nonetheless important step toward
identifying heart and blood vessel diseases or the potential for them. Although the history and exam by themselves usually do not offer a precise
diagnosis, they can suggest the need for additional tests and supply a
baseline to evaluate future changes in the health of patients.

During a routine physical, a nurse checks the temperature, pulse, and
blood pressure of the patient. Abnormalities in any of these indicators

may suggest heart or blood vessel problems. The physician obtains a medical history that includes questions about chest pain, leg pain with walking, weakness, shortness of breath, fluid buildup in the body, diet, exercise, smoking habits, and family history of heart disease—all symptoms or risk factors of heart disease. The physician also listens to the heart with a stethoscope placed at various positions on the body where the actions of each heart valve and chamber can be best heard. Sounds made by blood moving through the heart and blood vessels may point to heart valve problems and other forms of heart and blood vessel disease. Listening to the lungs as well as the heart can identify the presence of fluid, which often results from heart disease. Other assessments of skin color, swelling of the ankles, the size of the liver, the movement of blood through veins in the neck, the pulse in a variety of arteries, and other body characteristics supplement the information gained from listening to the heart and lungs. Even viewing the inside of the eye with a special instrument gives insight, as the clues to and consequences of heart and blood vessel abnormalities can show in the retina and tiny blood vessels. With all the information at hand, the physician can offer a clean bill of health, suggest lifestyle changes to prevent the emergence of problems, or suggest additional tests to obtain more information about possible heart and blood vessel problems.

### Blood Tests

Like the health history and physical exam, routine blood tests alone cannot diagnosis the existence of heart disease (although some special tests can identify whether those having chest pain are experiencing a heart attack). Rather, they identify high levels of substances in the blood that promote heart disease. To identify blood lipids or fats, tests check for levels of cholesterol, HDL, LDL, and triglycerides. In addition, tests can show the amount of time the blood takes to clot, the levels of blood materials that may lead to clotting, the functioning of the kidneys and liver, the presence of infection, and the amounts of minerals such as iron that increase the risk of heart disease. With such information, the physician can suggest changes in lifestyle, other tests for heart problems, and sometimes, medication to lower excess blood lipids.

The American Heart Association provides a checklist for lipid levels that guide doctors and patients in interpreting the results of blood tests.[4]

- For total cholesterol, levels less than 200 mg/dL are desirable, levels from 200 to 239 are borderline high and raise the risk of developing heart disease, and levels of 240 and above are high and double the risk of heart disease compared to someone with normal levels.

- For HDL, or good cholesterol, higher amounts are better than lower amounts. Levels less than 40 mg/dL increase the risk for developing heart disease, levels between 40 and 59 improve the risk, and levels 60 and above protect against the risk.

- The total cholesterol divided by the HDL offers a summary measure of blood lipids. A ratio less than five signifies positive lipid levels. The chances of a heart attack are low when total cholesterol falls below 200 mg/dL and HDL cholesterol exceeds 40 mg/dL.

- For LDL, or bad cholesterol, levels less than 129 mg/dL are desirable, levels from 130 to 159 are borderline high, and levels 160 and above are high. A low level of LDL corresponds to a low ratio of total cholesterol to HDL and also protects against the risk of heart disease.

- For triglycerides, blood levels do less well than cholesterol to predict heart problems but can provide helpful information. Levels of triglycerides less than 150 mg/dL are normal, levels from 150 to 199 are borderline high, levels from 200 to 499 are high, and levels 500 and above are very high.

Of course, these levels need to be interpreted in context. The presence of other risks for heart disease such as smoking, diabetes, high blood pressure, and a family history of heart problems makes high cholesterol levels all the more serious. In these cases, doctors will often recommend immediate treatment involving a change in diet and use of cholesterol-lowering drugs.

In recent years, doctors have started to measure the level of C-reactive protein along with blood lipids. This protein increases with inflammation, and high levels in the blood may stem from infection-caused swelling of vessels that can lead to blockages in the coronary arteries. High levels (3.0 mg/dL and above) indicate high risk for heart problems. For example, a study of women followed for eight years suggests that "C-reactive protein level is a stronger predictor of cardiovascular events than LDL cholesterol level and that it adds prognostic information."[5] Specifically, those in the upper third of scores for blood levels of the C-reactive protein have a risk of having a heart attack more than twice as high as those in the lower third of scores for blood levels of the protein. Although widely available, the tests are not used as routinely as cholesterol tests because the treatment appropriate for inflammation problems is less clear. The inflammation may reflect some form of infection, and antibiotics may help reduce the inflammation, but the benefits of such therapy have not been conclusively demonstrated. More research on causes, consequences, and treatment of blood vessel inflammation continues. In the meantime, the C-reactive protein test is reserved for those with a very high global risk assessment of heart disease.[6]

Blood tests reveal yet other information. Speedy clotting of the blood and high levels of substances that promote blood clotting reflect the potential for a blood clot to block delivery of blood to the heart. High levels of iron in the blood, according to some studies, also predict heart disease, and some doctors consider tests for iron in the blood to provide essential information.[7] However, the American Heart Association calls for more research on understanding iron's role in causing heart disease before screening patients on that basis and does not recommend reducing dietary levels of this crucial mineral.[8]

The nonroutine use of blood tests can determine if a person experiencing chest pain is having a heart attack. When parts of the muscle are injured or die because of the inability of blood, oxygen, and nutrients to get through the coronary arteries, certain cardiac enzymes leak into the blood. Some enzymes are released earlier in the injury process than others, and some stay longer in the blood than others. By measuring the presence of these various enzymes, doctors can determine the occurrence and timing of a heart attack.

## CONTROVERSY OVER CHOLESTEROL SCREENING

How young should people be when they first have their blood cholesterol levels checked? In some ways, it makes sense to screen for high cholesterol in young adulthood and perhaps even childhood—well before the risk of death from heart disease occurs. Since high cholesterol in youth and childhood may contribute to the long-term buildup of plaque in the coronary arteries that leads to heart attacks in adulthood, it suggests the need to check cholesterol levels at young ages. Then, early treatment can begin with lifestyle changes and cholesterol-lowering drugs. Guidelines thus recommend cholesterol testing every five years for adults starting at age 20,[9] and many public health officials push for similar screening of children and youth.[10]

However, in 1996, a report from the American College of Physicians, a professional group representing more than 85,000 internists, called for restricting routine testing of cholesterol.[11] According to the report, screening for high cholesterol among those without symptoms of heart disease should be limited to men ages 35 to 65 and women ages 45 to 65—the ages of highest risk for early death from heart disease. The authors of the report argue that medical research has not demonstrated the benefits of screening at younger and older ages. For young people, the report concludes: "Early treatment of high cholesterol in low-risk groups may not improve outcomes."[12] Drugs used to treat high cholesterol, for example, have not been tested in young people, and their long-term safety is unknown. Their use brings benefits to those with symptoms of coronary heart disease or those at ages when the underlying risks of a heart attack are greatest. But for younger people, these drugs may, given their unknown long-term side effects, do more harm than good. Even reducing cholesterol through diet may do little to reduce the risk of a heart attack when those risks are already quite low. At older ages as well, the evidence on the benefits of cholesterol-lowering therapy remains uncertain. In short, the report recommends waiting to screen for cholesterol when treatment will be most effective.

If screening for cholesterol among young adults brings little benefit, then screening among children and teens would do even less. Some suggest that cholesterol levels in children serve as poor predictors of cholesterol in young adulthood and are even poorer predictors of coronary heart disease in middle age.[13] In their view, the extra financial costs of paying for the early screening of children and the unnecessary worry created by the discovery of elevated levels of cholesterol warrant waiting until older ages for this test.

However, the American Heart Association calls proposals to limit screening to those in middle age incorrect and misguided.[14] To support their view, critics of the proposal cite a recent study that finds early screening can identify those at high risk of having a heart attack in decades to come. The study examined several large samples of men who were tested for cholesterol at ages 18–39 and followed for at least 16 years and up to 34 years to check for morality from heart disease.[15] Young men in the study with cholesterol levels higher than 200 mg/dL multiplied their risk of coronary heart disease by factors ranging from 2.15 to 3.63 and lowered their life expectancy from 3.8 to 8.7 years. By suggesting that early efforts to identify and treat high cholesterol bring benefits, these findings affirm the guidelines recommending that screening begin at age 20. Supporters of early screening further argue that drugs to lower cholesterol may work less well on someone who has already developed severe heart disease than on younger people at the early stages of the disease. Even if it does not lead to use of medication, early screening can help educate the young population about the risks of high cholesterol and lead them to pay more attention to nutrition, food labels, and healthy eating. The fact that a decline in population cholesterol levels occurred during decades when screening became widespread supports this claim.

The logic of the argument for early screening extends to childhood.[16] Pediatricians should, for example, check the cholesterol of children whose parents have high cholesterol, since the children may share the diet, activity levels, and genetic traits of parents.[17] High cholesterol levels in children may not warrant medication but can lead to efforts to improve diet and activity level. One study found that a change to skim milk from whole milk and to consumption of vegetable fat from saturated fat reduced cholesterol among children during their first few years of life.[18] Since atherosclerosis can begin in childhood—autopsies of teens reveal the early stages of the disease—efforts to lower cholesterol in children with particularly high levels may have long-term benefits.

To settle the controversy, researchers need to complete more long-term studies of the links of cholesterol levels in middle adulthood to levels in childhood and young adulthood, on the ability of young people to change their diet and physical activity in ways that reduce cholesterol, and on the long-term benefits and risks of cholesterol-lowering medications. In the meantime, it appears that efforts to screen early for high cholesterol will likely expand.

## ADVANCED METHODS OF DIAGNOSIS

### Chest X-Ray

A chest x-ray involves a simple test that can identify certain problems such as congestive heart failure and heart valve dysfunction. In general terms, the test involves taking special pictures of x-rays sent through the body. The penetration of the x-rays varies with the density of the body tissue; dense materials such as bone absorb more radiation and appear whiter on the resulting picture than less-dense materials. However, for body parts to show on the x-rays, the densities have to differ at the boundaries. For example, since the heart muscle and blood have similar densities, x-rays do not delineate them. More helpfully, x-rays may show if any of the heart valves are calcified and likely operating ineffectively, if the heart is enlarged by congestive heart failure, and if the lungs contain fluid resulting from the weak pumping ability of the heart. In these cases, different densities of the calcified valves compared with the surrounding tissue, of the heart compared with the adjacent lungs, and of the fluid compared with surrounding lung tissue make the chest x-ray a helpful diagnostic tool.

### Electrocardiogram and Stress Test

Abbreviated as ECG (or EKG, from the original Dutch version of the word), an electrocardiogram records the strength and patterns of electrical activity of the heart after electrodes are positioned on each arm and leg and on six spots on the chest. Each electrode is attuned to a different part of the heart and, with no pain to the patient, monitors the electrical impulses. Abnormal rhythms in the heartbeat will appear on the ECG, but so will some heart problems caused by inadequate blood and oxygen supply to parts of the heart that have been damaged during a heart attack. Problems related to high blood pressure, inherited electrical abnormalities, and cardiomyopathy can similarly appear on the ECG. In brief, damaged tissue does not generate normal electrical activity. The ECG provides a wealth of other information about the heart and remains one of the simplest but most important diagnostic tools in cardiology. An ECG even proves helpful in life-threatening situations: emergency ambulance personnel can transmit the ECG over the phone from the emergency scene or as they proceed toward the hospital. This lets emergency room physicians know what to expect when the ambulance arrives and even gives guidance to the paramedics about immediate treatment.

The diagnostic ability of an ECG improves when the heart is stressed by exercise rather than when beating at the normal rate. Although the most severe problems show when the heart is at rest and receives a normal supply of blood, other problems can remain hidden. An exercise stress test (or exercise tolerance test) involves monitoring the heart rate, ECG, and blood pressure as a patient gradually increases his or her physical activity on a treadmill or stationary bicycle until the heart rate reaches a target of about 85 percent of maximum. If the person cannot exercise, then medications can stress the heart without exercise. In either case, the exercise or pharmacological medication stress test can reveal problems in the electrical activity of the heart that otherwise might not appear. Since the exertion or medication can in rare instances (one out of five thousand) cause a heart attack or death, medical personnel carefully monitor and supervise the test.

A problem with ECGs is that they may occasionally produce false positives or apparent abnormalities in people without any heart disease. When used to screen otherwise healthy people, a positive test requires additional checks to affirm the indication of heart disease. The results of the test should, in other words, be used in combination with other information such as blood pressure, heart rate, and symptoms during and after the exercise or medication.

Sometimes an ECG in a lab or during the stress of exercise or medication does not last long enough to capture irregular heart rhythms that occur only occasionally. A Holter monitor records electrical activity of the heart while a person goes through normal daily activities and is particularly useful in identifying the occurrence of premature ventricular contractions. One simply wears a small tape recorder around the waist that is attached to electrodes on the body; the continuous record of electrical signals is analyzed later and used by the doctor to identify various types of heart arrhythmia. In some cases, patient-activated recorders are useful for capturing episodes of heart irregularities.

### Echocardiogram

An echocardiogram uses an ultrasound beam or sound wave to view the heart in motion (much as a fetus is viewed before birth). Usually done by placing a small instrument on the chest, an echocardiogram in some cases involves inserting the instrument into the mouth and down the esophagus so that its closeness to the heart produces more detailed images. The images can identify enlargement of the heart, abnormal motion of the muscular walls of the heart, abnormal fluid collected in the sac around the heart, and problems in the functioning of heart valves, but most often they help identify abnormalities in the motion of the heart muscle that may result from the lack of sufficient blood. Abnormalities in the motion of the heart wall can reveal coronary heart disease, locate the probable region of the coronary artery responsible for a heart attack, and survey the damage done by a heart attack. An echocardiogram usually cannot provide a direct image of the coronary arteries themselves but improves on the ability of an ECG to diagnose coronary heart disease. Like a stress ECG test, an echocardiogram after exercise or medication often reveals hidden problems in the motion of the heart wall.

### Nuclear Imaging Techniques

Nuclear imaging techniques reverse the use of an x-ray. Instead of sending radioactive waves through the body, a radioactive substance is injected into the body, and special cameras observe the movement of the substance through the heart and related structures. The radioactive substances used in nuclear imaging decay quickly and remain in the blood only long enough for the test. Depending on the particular type of nuclear scanning technique used, the resulting images allow cardiologists to diagnose several possible heart problems.

First, in radionuclide ventriculography, a tiny amount of a radioisotope injected into the bloodstream is measured when it passes through the left ventricle, the chamber responsible for sending oxygen-rich blood to the body. The percentage of blood ejected from the left ventricle (called the ejection fraction) is normally about 60 percent and indicates severe weakness and high risk for future problems when less than 45 percent.

Second, in a perfusion scan, the injected radioactive material is absorbed by healthy heart tissue, but damaged heart tissue, because it receives less blood, absorbs the material more slowly. Particularly useful when it follows a stress test, this scan can help determine the regions of blocked coronary arteries. Parts of the heart that do not receive the radioactive material because of damage will show up immediately. A second scan performed four hours later can distinguish between heart muscle temporarily blocked from receiving blood and oxygen from heart muscle permanently blocked. If defects have disappeared, it indicates exercise or medication-induced ischemia; if the defects persist, it indicates permanent scarring. This part of the test helps determine how much of the heart has been permanently damaged by a heart attack.

### Computed Tomography

Although not often recommended to diagnose heart disease, computed tomography (CT or CAT) provides a three-dimensional picture of the heart that can help disclose some types of abnormalities and their exact location. Rather than scanning for the movement and location of radioactive material, the procedure measures the weakening of x-rays after they have passed through the body tissue. As an x-ray tube rotates around the body, the x-ray beams are detected after they have passed through the body, and the information is relayed to a computer for creating an image. Completely painless and noninvasive, the scan focuses on problems involving the structure of the heart muscle and the major vessels leading to and from the heart. A variation on the standard procedure called an electron beam computed tomography or ultrafast CT detects calcification in the coronary arteries, but its effectiveness in identifying coronary heart disease remains unclear.

## THE MARKETING OF CT SCANS

CAT Scan 2000, a Florida company with mobile units that travel across the country, offers ultrafast CT heart scans for only $199.[19] In widely marketing the procedure, the company proudly calls itself the Wal-Mart of scanning. The company and others like it promise to provide an early warning of heart disease among adults without any symptoms. If those with abnormalities identified by the scan get treatment for their problem, it can prevent premature and unexpected death. Ads further highlight the easy, quick, and painless nature of the procedure. The scan is seldom recommended by physicians or paid for by insurance but has become popular as private businesses market it over radio and television. The problem, according to critics, is that the scan can find something wrong with nearly everyone and often cannot distinguish between minor problems that do not threaten health and major problems that do. In relation to heart disease, signs of calcification in the coronary arteries that the scan identifies do not inevitably mean serious disease. If the ultrafast CT scan unnecessarily leads to more expensive tests and anxiety, it does more harm than good. Dr. William Casarella, after having a scan that suggested several problems involving cancer, went through $47,000 worth of further tests to find out that the scan identified benign abnormalities.[20] Applied to heart disease and other diagnoses, the excessive use of scans can lead to incorrect diagnoses. At the same time, however, some physicians think that the ultrafast CT scan should be studied and, if used appropriately, can in the future bring benefits in diagnosing heart disease. Once large clinical trials validate the diagnosis technique and bring it into the mainstream, such scans may offer advantages over more invasive diagnostic procedures.[21]

### Magnetic Resonance Imaging

Rather than using x-rays or injected radioactive materials, magnetic resonance imaging (MRI) uses magnetic fields and radio waves to obtain detailed images of the structures of the heart. Patients are placed inside a large electromagnet that causes atomic nuclei in the body to vibrate and give out signals that are converted into images of cardiac structures. Because the technique does better than others to distinguish blood from soft tissue, it can provide exceptionally detailed images of the heart wall, valves, and vessels. New forms of the procedure include coronary magnetic resonance imaging, which may reveal atherosclerosis by depicting blood at the site of a proximal narrowing of the coronary arteries in different hues than blood flowing more smoothly.[22]

### Cardiac Catheterization and Angiography

The most invasive but also the most accurate procedure for diagnosing coronary artery heart disease and other heart problems involves using a catheter or long tube. The catheter is inserted into an artery or vein of the leg or arm and is advanced to the heart. This cardiac catheterization procedure takes place in the hospital, where the patient receives local anesthesia and a mild sedative. The doctors use continuous x-ray images to guide and monitor the progress of the catheter. Once in the heart, the catheter can measure blood pressure in the ventricles and major arteries, as well as the flow of blood through and out of the heart. If the pressure appears too low or high, it indicates problems in the functioning of the valves, ventricles, and lungs. If the blood flow falls below normal, less blood gets to the body, and more oxygen has to be extracted from the blood.

Most often, however, the cardiac catheterization procedure is used to perform a contrast angiography. A special dye or contrast agent is injected into the heart through the catheter, and x-ray exposures of the contrast agent record a moving image or angiogram of the heart. When the contrast agent is injected into the heart chamber, the angiogram helps identify heart valve problems, abnormal thickening of the muscle wall, blood clots in the heart, and congenital malformations. More commonly, the dye is injected through the catheter directly into the coronary arteries rather than the heart. Called a coronary artery angiography, the method pinpoints the existence and location of any blockages in the coronary arteries that limit the flow of blood to the heart muscle. If many blockages appear, they may require heart bypass surgery. More often, blowing up a small balloon at the site of the blockage (called angioplasty) can reduce the blockage, and propping open the artery (using a stent) can prevent the blockage from recurring.

Although it is the best procedure for diagnosing coronary heart disease and other problems in the structure and function of the heart, cardiac catheterization is also the most risky. In rare cases (about one out of a thousand), the procedure can cause heart attacks, strokes, abnormal heart rhythms, and even death. The procedure itself does not cause the patient much pain, but the possibility of an adverse heart event requires that it be done in the hospital and under the close supervision and monitoring of physicians.

## THE FIRST HEART CATHETERIZATION

In 1929, Werner Forssmann, a German physician fresh out of medical school, provided a way to see into the heart. Forssmann wanted to be able to deliver drugs directly to the heart in an emergency but knew that injecting them through the blind insertion of a needle into the chest created undue risk of error. He reasoned that since the veins send blood back to the heart, they must provide a pathway to the heart (or more specifically, the right atrium of the heart). Experimenting with cadavers, he found he could insert a long narrow tube or catheter into a vein in front of the elbow all the way to the heart. Wanting to try the technique on a living person but unwilling to subject a patient to possible harm, he decided to perform the catheterization on himself. In so doing, he had to disregard orders of his supervisors. Not surprisingly, they viewed the idea of pushing a long tube through the body and into the heart as a crazy experiment and had forbidden it.

Proceeding anyway, Forssmann injected a small amount of anesthetic into his arm, made a small incision in the skin, inserted a narrow tube into his arm, pushed the tube about a foot inside, and took an x-ray picture of his arm to see how far the tube had gone. However, at this moment, a colleague came into the room, became angry at what he saw, and called Forssmann an idiot. Forssmann wrote that his colleague "nearly tried to pull the catheter out of my arm. I had to give him a few kicks on the shin to calm him down." Forssmann then bravely (or recklessly) pushed the catheter two feet in—to inside the heart—without harm. An x-ray picture documented this accomplishment. The publication of the film and the description of the procedure caused a sensation. Several colleagues called the procedure a circus trick, and others found the idea of inserting a tube through the body and into the heart disgusting.

Despite such criticism, Forssmann continued his experiments. The next step involved injecting a substance through the catheter and into the heart. Because the substance contained iodine, it could be seen with x-rays as it moved through a pumping heart. He found that the substance could safely be inserted into the hearts of dogs but would kill rabbits. To check on the procedure for humans, he again served as the experimental subject. After inserting the catheter and injecting the substance into the heart chamber, he experienced no ill effects, but his inferior x-ray equipment took poor pictures. A few years later, two physicians, André F. Cournand and Dickinson W. Richards, Jr., helped perfect the technique, and all three shared the Nobel Prize in Medicine in 1956.[23] In the late 1950s, researchers further discovered that the contrast agent could be injected into the coronary arteries as well as into the heart without harm to the patient.

## BENEFITS OF EARLY DIAGNOSIS AND IDENTIFICATION OF RISK

Primary prevention aims to thwart the development of heart disease in persons without any symptoms, while secondary prevention aims to protect patients who already have heart disease. Secondary prevention is, in one sense, more efficient because it focuses on those most in need of help and treats fewer patients to save a life. However, secondary prevention works best with early diagnosis and early medical intervention Waiting to treat heart disease until it leads to a heart attack or debilitating angina pain risks the death of the patient and creates problems for doctors in rectifying a disease at advanced stages. Techniques to improve the ability to diagnose heart disease early can make medical interventions more effective.

Health histories and physical exams, blood pressure, pulse rate, heart rhythm measures, cholesterol checks, and ECGs can provide preliminary evidence of a problem and lead to initial, often quite effective means to deal with the problem. Although not identical to heart disease, both high blood pressure and high cholesterol levels increase the risk of developing or worsening the disease. The early indication of high risk can lead doctors to recommend changes in dietary and exercise habits or to prescribe medications. Such steps may prevent any existing disease from progressing any further than it has and even induce regression of the disease.

More sophisticated tests can help identify patients with hidden heart problems. For example, siblings of people with heart disease are known to have a high risk for heart attacks, but the usual tests often cannot detect a problem. In a study of more than seven hundred people ages 30 to 59 with a brother or sister who had heart disease, the subjects were given a stress test and then also injected with a radioactive dye near the end of a workout and examined with a two-dimensional nuclear imaging device to measure blood flow. The nuclear imaging method found previously undiagnosed heart disease in about 20 percent of the subjects.[24]

In addition to helping to identify the existence of heart problems, diagnostic techniques can identify the specific source of the problem. Chest x-rays, ECGs, blood tests, echocardiograms, nuclear imaging methods, CT scans, and MRI scans provide detailed information on the specific nature of heart disease and help doctors devise treatment regimes to prevent early death from the disease. Continued diagnostic testing can then measure the success of the treatment in dealing with heart disease, disclose lack of progress and the need for changes in the regimes, and improve the search for better treatment. If cardiology once required much guesswork, technology today shines light (figuratively) on the abnormal operation of the heart.

Knowing the site of coronary artery blockages proves particularly helpful before making a decision to perform angioplasty, insertion of stents, or heart surgery—a serious, expensive, and sometimes life-threatening procedure. Coronary artery angiograms can identify the locations and determine the seriousness of blockages in the coronary arteries. If bypass surgery appears necessary to deal with the blockages, the angiogram lets surgeons know what they will face in the surgery. Information gained from other diagnostic tests about valve problems also aids in other forms of heart surgery. Much as a general going into battle wants to know the strength of the enemy, a surgeon wants to know what to expect when doing heart surgery. Accurate diagnostic techniques can thus improve the success of the surgery and help extend the life of patients.

For people experiencing chest pain, a blood test can now quickly reveal if the pain is caused by a heart attack and requires immediate treatment (unlike what happened to President Eisenhower during his heart attack when such blood tests did not exist). Chest pain is common but often is not due to heart disease. The diagnostic ability allows physicians to distinguish cases that require immediate heart treatment from cases that require referral to a gastroenterologist or psychiatrist rather than a cardiologist.[25]

## PROGRESS IN DIAGNOSIS

Many of the diagnostic techniques used today are relatively new or are used in new, more effective ways. The advances in diagnostic procedures thus correspond to the reductions in heart disease mortality and likely played an important role in the reductions. In the 1970s, only a few tests were available to identify the nature and extent of heart disease: ECG, chest x-ray, and blood tests. Since then, numerous tests have emerged. "In the ten year period between 1975 and 1984, there was a dramatic increase in the use of a wide variety of diagnostic procedures in patients hospitalized with AMI [acute myocardial infarction]."[26] From 1980 to 1990, figures suggest that about 70 percent of the drop in deaths from coronary artery disease resulted from treatment of patients with heart disease: "Most of the decline was explained by improvements in the management of patients with diagnosed CHD [coronary heart disease] through risk factor reduction and improvements in treatment."[27] Given this improvement, allowing patients to receive medical treatment is the key to diagnosis of coronary heart disease.

Consider three examples of how increased use of diagnostic tests likely contributed to progress against heart disease. First, cholesterol screening has grown so much that a large majority of adults now have had a test in the last five years (as is recommended by national guidelines). In 1999, the Behavioral Risk Factor Surveillance System interviewed by telephone a randomly selected sample of adults ages 18 and over in 47 states.[28] The survey measured whether respondents had a blood cholesterol test in the past five years. According to the responses, the median having had the test across the states was 72 percent. Maryland had the highest screening with 79.2 percent, and Minnesota had the lowest with 57.5 percent. Room for improvement remains, and progress in recent years has slowed, but the 72 percent figure contrasts with the rarity of such tests several decades ago.

Second, screening for high blood pressure has led to the widespread treatment of hypertension—a problem particularly severe in minority communities. In the late 1960s and early 1970s, the situation with regard to hypertension was not encouraging: about half the cases of high blood pressure remained undetected.[29] Since the launching of the National High Blood Pressure Education Program in 1973, the majority of persons with high blood pressure—including those from more disadvantaged groups and parts of the country—have been identified (and treated). As a result, the proportion of the population with high blood pressure has declined. The treatment of hypertension may have explained, according to some estimates, about 8.5 to 17 percent of the decline in coronary mortality rates between 1968 and 1976.[30]

Third, a study of treatment of those hospitalized for heart attacks in Minneapolis–St. Paul from 1985 to 1995 found that the use of angiography increased from 22 to 59 percent for men and 18 to 57 percent for women.[31] The use of echocardiography increased from 35 to 55 percent for men and 36 to 65 percent for women. Consistent with the use of these tests in the hospital, the study further found that heart attack incidents and deaths from heart disease in the hospital declined substantially during the period.

Overall, then, greater use of both older and newer diagnostic techniques has helped identify those with heart disease and determine the individual treatment most appropriate for a patient. This progress in diagnostic ability has contributed to the fall in heart disease mortality, although exact figures on the contribution are difficult to estimate. The major concern about the widespread use of diagnostic testing is financial rather than medical. The more advanced tests are expensive and may clash with medical cost control measures. For example, a stress test costs about $250, while a nuclear imaging perfusion test costs about $1,000.[32] With the Medicare system facing future bankruptcy, private health insurance fees rising, and health maintenance organizations (HMOs) facing financial pressures, cost containment efforts may require special emphasis on cost-effective diagnosis. For example, physicians may need to limit screening tests to those who appear at high risk for developing heart disease rather than offering the tests to all adults. At the same time, insurance companies may recognize that early diagnosis—even if expensive—saves money if it prevents even more expensive surgery. Such debates will continue but do not negate the importance of diagnosis for the progress made against heart disease.

# CHAPTER 4

# Treatment of Heart Disease

In 1954, Norman Cousins, who would become a nationally known magazine editor and author of the best-selling *Anatomy of an Illness*, had undergone a life insurance exam that included an electrocardiogram. When the insurance doctors found evidence of an earlier heart attack in the test, they recommended that Cousins give up his job, sports activity, and travel and take to bed.[1] In 1955, Lyndon Johnson, then the powerful Senate majority leader, later the vice president under President John F. Kennedy, and still later the president himself, had a heart attack. After thinking it was indigestion and taking an anti-acid and some whiskey for the pain, he was sent to the hospital, where he went into severe shock and remained in critical condition for several days.[2] The recommended treatment for the serious heart condition? Six weeks in the hospital and three months of complete rest at home. Both Cousins and Johnson fortunately lived decades longer, but the treatment regimes at the time seem in retrospect to be primitive.

Dr. Isadore Rosenfeld, writing in *Parade Magazine*, notes that when he was in medical school decades ago, "There was little that a cardiologist could do for someone who'd had a heart attack other than to interpret the electrocardiogram, prescribe prolonged bed rest and offer tender loving care."[3] That treatment may have in fact created new problems: "We kept such patients flat on their backs for six weeks, leaving them vulnerable to the formation of blood clots, which often traveled to a lung artery, causing pulmonary embolism and death."[4]

Contrast the treatment of Cousins and Johnson some 40 to 50 years ago with someone who received modern treatment for his heart problems. In

1988, Max Kramer, a sociologist whose research specialized in the productivity of members of a work team, experienced dizziness, severe sweating, and a pain in his right arm and shoulder.[5] His wife drove him to a clinic where, after an examination, the doctors said he was having a heart attack and needed emergency hospital treatment. Loaded on an ambulance and monitored by paramedics, Kramer reached the hospital less than an hour after the first symptoms started. At the hospital, he received a clot-busting drug and watched on a TV monitor with the medical team as the drug dissolved the clot causing the heart attack. Everyone in the room cheered. Next, the head of the medical team performed a balloon angioplasty. Kramer could again watch as a thin wire wound its way to the heart and into the coronary artery where the balloon expanded and widened the narrow spot in the artery. Some 10 years later, despite improving his lifestyle with exercise and a better diet and undergoing heart bypass surgery, Kramer received news of having congestive heart failure. Fluid in his lungs had built up because the heart had weakened to the point where it could no longer pump well enough to remove the fluid. This time, treatment through the prescription of new beta-blocker drugs and diuretics rectified the problem.

David Moses, age 88 in 1999, has lived with heart disease for 34 years and seen personally how the treatment for heart disease has changed dramatically.[6] In 1965 at age 54, chest pain led to a diagnosis of angina, but the cardiologists merely prescribed nitroglycerin tablets that, when taken on the occurrence of chest pain, would relax the coronary arteries and temporarily relieve the angina symptoms. His doctors did not even tell him to stop smoking, as knowledge of the harm of the habit for heart health was not fully understood. In decades to come, however, Moses started to receive more aggressive treatment in response to worsening of his symptoms. In 1978, he underwent heart bypass surgery; in 1986, the cardiologist put him on cholesterol-lowering drugs; in 1996, surgery repaired an aneurysm in his aorta; in 1997, he had a pacemaker inserted to regulate the beating of his heart; and in 1998, he had stents put into coronary arteries to help keep them from narrowing. Moses nicely summarizes his experiences:

So here I am in 1999, thirty-four years after first developing angina, with a body that is walking testimony to modern medical procedures and devices: five grafts to bypass my blocked coronary arteries, a plastic tube in place of part of my aorta, a pacemaker that beats my heart for me whenever necessary, and three stents to widen my narrowed coronary arteries. Without all this technology I would have died long ago.[7]

Technology alone does not fully account for Moses's longevity—he also started consuming a low-fat diet and exercising regularly to improve his health—but it played an essential role.

Compared with the experiences of Norman Cousins and Lyndon Johnson, those of Max Kramer and David Moses reveal the enormous progress made in treating heart disease. Millions of other persons have benefited from new treatment regimes and lived longer, healthier, and richer lives because of modern medicine. This chapter reviews the medications and minor surgical procedures used today to treat persons with diagnosed heart disease (the next chapter reviews major surgical procedures such as heart bypass surgery).

Before beginning the review, however, recall the varied types of heart problems that need treatment:

- Coronary artery disease, the major cause of ischemia (lack of oxygen for the heart muscle), angina (chest pain), and myocardial infarction (heart attack), involves blockages in the coronary arteries that obstruct the flow of blood and oxygen to the heart muscle.

- Heart failure stems from a variety of sources, including coronary artery disease, but involves the weakening of the heart muscle such that blood does not adequately circulate through the body and water retention swells parts of the body.

- Heart valve disease involves the narrowing (stenosis) of the valves between the heart chambers such that blood cannot flow fully from one chamber to the other, or improper closing (regurgitation) such that the blood flows back after it passes from one chamber to another.

- Heart rhythm problems involve the irregular beating of the heart.

- Long QT syndrome presents a risk of sudden death.

- High cholesterol and high blood pressure, although not heart disease themselves, increase the risks of several types of heart disease.

Some medications help treat multiple heart problems, while others are specific to one type of problem. Consider some of the most commonly used ones.[8]

## HEART MEDICATIONS

### Aspirin

Aspirin helps lower the risk of a recurrence for those who have already had a heart attack or stroke. It also helps those with unstable angina, which involves frequent and intense pain and usually results from a blood clot in a coronary artery. Aspirin (including some super-aspirins prescribed for heart disease rather than aches and pains) makes the blood less sticky so as to reduce the likelihood of this harmful clotting process. Early evidence of the benefits for men has now been supplemented by evidence that it benefits women.[9]

Nonetheless, the U.S. Food and Drug Administration has not approved aspirin for preventing heart attacks in healthy individuals.[10] Although it can lower the risk of a heart attack by helping to keep the arteries open and make the blood less sticky, aspirin can also have some negative effects. It can cause stomach bleeding, bleeding in the brain, kidney failure, and some kinds of strokes. It can also lead to more severe problems if the patient already uses other medications to thin blood. Use of low-dose or baby aspirin instead of regular aspirin minimizes these problems. Still, the potential for harmful side effects suggests the need for careful discussion of the use of aspirin by patient and doctor.

## Warfarin

Heart failure and sluggish blood flow can promote the formation of clots in the heart chamber and leg veins. If the clot breaks off and travels through the bloodstream, it can cause a stroke or other serious complications. Blood thinners such as warfarin are therefore used for persons with heart failure or atrial fibrillation. Warfarin acts by preventing the liver from using vitamin K to produce clotting proteins, but its use requires tests of the clotting time of the blood to determine dosage. Other anticoagulants may also be helpful. For example, when administered intravenously for hospitalized patients, heparin reduces blood clotting.

## Digitalis

One of the oldest medications available, digitalis derives from the foxglove plant and was first used more than two hundred years ago. By making the heart contract harder and slowing down an excessively rapid heart pulse, this medication helps those with congestive heart failure and weakening of the heart's pumping function. It can also help those whose hearts are impaired by valve disease or by atrial fibrillation. Other similar medications offer immediate help for those with serious heart failure when used intravenously. However, despite its ability to improve symptoms and reduce hospitalizations from heart failure, digitalis does not appear to improve survival.[11]

---

### A FOLK REMEDY BECOMES A HEART MEDICATION

Although enormous advances have occurred in the development of medications for heart disease in the last decade or two, digitalis was used for centuries as a natural remedy of heart disease—and is still used today.[12] Congestive heart failure or cardiac edema has afflicted persons throughout history with painful swelling of the legs and loss of energy. Historically, it was called dropsy. Going back to at least the thirteenth century, peasants of western Europe had discovered that the powdered leaves of a wild plant with lovely purple flowers shaped like bells brought relief to those suffering from dropsy. The plant had the formal name, *Digitalis purpurea,* or the purple foxglove. Although they did not understand how it worked, biologists in the sixteenth century recognized that it drew off water from the body and purified the blood.

Early medicine unfortunately did not take advantage of the folk knowledge. Some mistakenly recommended foxglove as a cure for epilepsy and tuberculosis, and others prescribed excessive—and toxic—amounts of the product. Foxglove became known as a powerful poison rather than a medication.

William Withering, the son of a famous English doctor and a graduate of Edinburgh University in Scotland with a degree in medicine, corrected this misunderstanding. Familiar with plants in England and hearing from an old woman about one plant that would help rid the body of unwanted fluid, Withering began to experiment with foxglove. His experiments produced remarkable results in one patient, Miss Hill of Aston, whose severe heart failure produced extreme shortness of breath. Withering describes the results of giving Miss Hill a liquid form of the foxglove plant: "[It] acted very powerfully on the kidneys, for within the first twenty-four hours she made upwards of eight quarts of water. The sense of fullness and oppression across her stomach was greatly diminished, her breath was eased, her pulse became more full and regular, and the swellings of her legs subsided."[13]

Withering published a book in 1785 describing his systematic observations over 10 years on the use of digitalis. The book prescribes the proper amount—the same amount used today—and warned against overuse. It also mentions that digitalis affected the heart, thus making the link between the heart and blood circulation problems at a time when understanding of human anatomy was just emerging. His work on the benefits of this medication for those with dropsy made Withering rich and famous. Even Benjamin Franklin consulted him by letter about treatment for his kidney stones. Withering may not have had much understanding about how his prescription worked, but he nonetheless made a lasting contribution to the treatment of heart disease.

## ACE (Angiotensin Converting Enzyme) Inhibitors

An alternative approach to dealing with heart failure aims to reduce the workload of the heart and make it more efficient rather than make it contract harder (as with digitalis). This can be done by widening the arteries through which the blood flows and lowering the resistance the blood pressure would have to work against. Much as forcing a liquid out of a squeeze bottle is easier when the opening is wide rather than narrow, pumping of blood can be done efficiently when the arteries are widened. Vasodilator drugs perform this function. One widely used class of vasodilators, ACE (angiotensin converting enzyme) inhibitors, decreases the production of a chemical, angiotensin II, that causes the blood vessels to constrict. By widening the vessels, ACE inhibitors help control high blood pressure. For those with damaged heart tissue from a heart attack, heart valve disease, or heart failure more generally, they allow the heart to pump more easily and efficiently and to better supply the body with blood. These medications both reduce symptoms and extend survival in patients.[14] A new class of blood pressure drugs called angiotensin antagonists shields blood vessels from angiotensin II and also helps deal with high blood pressure and heart failure.[15]

### Nitrates (Including Nitroglycerine)

Nitrates relax and dilate blood vessels. The effects of this action include (1) redistributing the blood from the heart chambers to the vessels and reducing the pressure on the heart chambers, (2) lowering the resistance the heart encounters in pumping blood into the arteries, and (3) increasing the blood that can flow through partially blocked coronary arteries.[16] One common form of nitrates, nitroglycerine, is taken by dissolving a pill under the tongue when experiencing angina pain. It quickly lessens the pain and symptoms of angina or coronary spasm—an abnormal tendency for the coronary arteries to constrict intermittently. Patients use it according to circumstances rather than continuously.

### Calcium Channel Blockers

Calcium channel blockers relax blood vessels, reduce blood pressure, and moderate chest pain by interrupting the normal flow of calcium to cells. The blockers thus dilate arteries, particularly the coronary arteries, and make it easier for the heart to pump blood through the body. They also reduce blood pressure, ease the oxygen demand of the heart, and normalize some types of irregular heart rhythms.

### Beta- (and Alpha-) Blockers

Beta-blockers help deal with blood pressure and heart problems by moderating the effect of norepinephrine, a hormone that may excite the heart. By slowing the heart and making it beat with less contracting force, beta-blockers reduce blood pressure and heart rate, the strain placed on the heart, and the heart's need for oxygen. They are prescribed for high blood pressure, angina, heart attack recovery, heart failure, and some irregular heart rhythms. A variation, alpha-beta-blockers, not only slows the heart but also reduces blood pressure by slowing nerve impulses to blood vessels and allowing the blood to flow more easily.

### Diuretics

Sometimes called water pills, diuretics eliminate fluid in the body and help treat high blood pressure and swelling from congestive heart failure. By promoting urine production in the kidneys, diuretics remove water and sodium from the body, which means fluid flows from tissue back into the bloodstream and swelling falls. They do not correct the problems causing heart failure but effectively deal with the side effects.[17]

### High Blood Pressure Drugs

Along with ACE inhibitors, calcium channel blockers, beta-blockers, and diuretics, many other drugs help treat hypertension. Some affect control centers in the brain, some act on the walls of the blood vessels, and some affect the vessel nerves, but all work to lower blood pressure and the associated risks for heart disease.

### Anti-Arrhythmia Drugs

Most anti-arrhythmia drugs treat a fast or irregular rhythm, but others can be given intravenously in emergency situations to speed up a slow heart rhythm. They work by altering the way electrical currents flow through the heart's conduction system and muscle. However, the medications can worsen rhythm disturbances in some patients and need to be carefully monitored. Since a large number of medications help deal with rhythm problems, some clinical testing is needed in every patient to find the proper product and dosage level for that patient.

### Thrombolytic Agents

Also called clot-busting drugs, thrombolytic agents are given during a heart attack to break up a blood clot in the coronary arteries and to restore blood flow. To be most effective and to prevent permanent damage to the heart, they need to be given within one hour of the start of the heart attack symptoms. Restoring blood flow as quickly as possible—something best done at the hospital—can do much to prevent a heart attack from causing death. Thrombolytics can be given intravenously or administered with a catheter inserted through the vessels. When targeted directly at the clot, these medications prove highly effective.

## BLOOD CHOLESTEROL–LOWERING AGENTS: STATINS

### A New Wonder Drug

Although consuming a healthful, low-fat diet represents the first step to controlling blood cholesterol levels, most people with atherosclerotic heart and blood vessel disease need more than a change in diet. A variety of medications can help lower cholesterol, but use of a relatively new class of drugs called statins has become particularly common. About 15 million Americans now take the drugs, and by some estimates, another 30–36 million people at risk of cardiovascular disease could benefit from taking them. The American Heart Association states, "It appears the widespread use of statins will be one of the most potent weapons we have in reducing the risk of Americans dying early of heart disease."[18] A cardiologist says of statins, "They are one of the most important advances in pharmacological therapy in any area of medicine over the past 20 years."[19] Some go so far as to call statins a "wonder drug."

---

### GOOD ENOUGH FOR PRESIDENTS

In the days before leaving office, President Bill Clinton was found during a routine physical to have elevated cholesterol. Both the president and the doctors did not see the higher level, which reached 233 mg/dL, as serious. President Clinton noted, "My cholesterol is a little too high because I haven't exercised and I ate all that Christmas dessert. But in six months it'll be back to normal." His doctor agreed that once out of office, the president would be better able to control his lifestyle. Still, he was given a prescription of the medication Zocor, a statin to reduce his blood cholesterol. With benefits of statins seeming to accrue even to those without heart disease, President Clinton joined millions of others taking the medication.[20]

---

### Benefits of Statins

Why such optimism? The drugs not only reduce the prevalence of LDL cholesterol in the blood but in so doing also reduce the risk of a heart attack. An overview of research trials found that statins lower total cholesterol by 22 percent and LDL cholesterol by 30 percent.[21] Another study found that statin drug treatment was associated with a 20 percent reduction in total cholesterol, a 28 percent reduction in LDL cholesterol, a 13 percent reduction in triglycerides, and a 5 percent increase in HDL cholesterol.[22] While reducing the bad LDL cholesterol, statins do not reduce the good HDL cholesterol. Those with very high cholesterol levels and serious heart disease can benefit most from such changes in blood lipids, but those with moderately elevated cholesterol levels and no symptoms of heart disease may also reduce their risk of developing the disease.

Corresponding to the improvements in blood makeup, cardiovascular mortality appears about 30 percent lower and total morality about 22 percent lower among those taking statins compared with a control group receiving a placebo.[23] Equally important, no evidence has emerged that there is an increase in other types of death such as strokes—to the contrary, death from many other causes declines with statins.[24] As one physician puts it, "These benefits are seen across this huge range of high-risk individuals—male, female, young, old—and irrespective of their cholesterol level. I think this will change the way we practice medicine in terms of reducing risk in these high-risk individuals."[25]

Statins may have other favorable effects besides lowering cholesterol. They appear to lessen C-reactive protein levels and modify inflammation that promotes coronary artery disease, to help prevent osteoporosis and bone problems, and to perhaps even reduce the risk of Alzheimer's disease.[26] By helping the flow of blood to the small blood vessels in the brain, statins may prevent brain atrophy and susceptibility to dementia. These initial findings need to be replicated with additional studies, but they are intriguing and contribute to the growing reputation of statins. Lastly, statins appear as an alternative to hormone replacement therapy for postmenopausal women. Initially thought to reduce the risk of heart disease, hormone therapy (including increased estrogen) was found in a government study to actually increase the risk of heart disease. This new finding suggests that women at risk of heart disease should use alternatives to hormone replacement therapy such as statins.[27]

Sold under the brand names Zocor, Lipitor, Lescol, Pravachol, Advicor, and Mevacor (Lovastatin in its generic form), statins have become the nation's second-most-prescribed class of drugs.[28] The U.S. government first approved their use in 1987, and since then they have been widely prescribed. Despite this popularity, doctors appear less willing to prescribe the medication than many experts would like, and patients appear less willing to comply with the treatment than doctors would like. Some estimate that only about one of five who could benefit from the products actually use them.[29] Doctors, being more used to treating disease rather than preventing it, seem hesitant to prescribe statins widely. They may have lingering concerns about safety and high cost ($50 to $135 a month).[30] Patients without symptoms of heart disease remain unconcerned about the problem. Although statins help protect them from harm in the future, patients do not feel better immediately when they take the medication (and may even experience some unpleasant side effects). Thus, some patients who receive a prescription simply do not comply. One researcher who has studied compliance states, "If you give it to patients, do they take the drug? The answer is a pretty emphatic, 'No.' "[31]

Besides being expensive, statins have side effects that sometimes become serious.[32] One statin, Baycol, was discontinued in 2001 after being linked to 31 deaths related to kidney failure. Less seriously, they can also cause muscle pain or weakness (myopathy) and liver irritation. Other long-term side effects, despite the use of statins for 15 years, will not yet be apparent. A review of the evidence suggests that severe muscle problems due to statins are extremely rare,[33] but the potential for problems suggests that statins should be used carefully. Doctors know what symptoms to watch for in patients on statins and can discontinue a medication that causes problems. Those who can gain from the use of statins should be concerned about side effects, but they should also be concerned about the high risk of death from heart disease that statins can reduce.

### How They Work

Statins reduce cholesterol in the blood by preventing the liver from producing its own cholesterol. Necessary for life, cholesterol is both manufactured in the liver and obtained directly from food. However, cholesterol for many is obtained in sufficient amounts through the diet to make production by the body unnecessary. Statins, or HMG-CoA reductase in scientific terms, block an enzyme in the liver that synthesizes cholesterol and prevent the liver from producing and releasing cholesterol in the blood stream.

The discovery of statins began in Japan as Akira Endo and his colleagues searched for new antibiotics.[34] Since the antibiotic penicillin was found in a mold that inhibited bacterial growth, the search for new antibiotics focused on funguses. Endo and colleagues knew that bacteria needed cholesterol to grow and hoped to isolate cholesterol-inhibiting HMG-CoA reductase to block the bacterial growth. They managed to isolate two such inhibitors, while others discovered similar forms. Researchers at pharmaceutical companies later developed them into products for cholesterol control that humans could use.

The understanding of the beneficial consequences of blocking liver production of cholesterol comes from the Nobel Prize–winning research of Michael Brown and Joseph Goldstein.[35] In 1973, they discovered a protein receptor on the surface of cells that grabs LDL—the carriers of cholesterol—out of the blood and pulls them inside for crucial cell functions. They further found that when a person has too few LDL receptors, cholesterol remains in the blood, reaches high levels, and can add to plaque formation on vessel walls. In rare cases, a genetically caused deficit in LDL receptors leads to extremely high levels of cholesterol in the blood and sometimes to severe heart disease in children and young adults. Under normal circumstances, however, receptors shuttle back and forth from the cell surface to inside the cell about once every 10 minutes.[36] When statins inhibit cholesterol synthesis in the liver, it triggers an increase in LDL receptors that reduces blood levels of LDL cholesterol. As the liver produces less of its own cholesterol, then, its capacity to snatch LDL cholesterol from the blood improves.

Other drugs that lower cholesterol work differently than statins.[37] Bile acid sequestrants bind with cholesterol in the intestines and eliminate it through the stool. Still other medications—nicotinic acid and fibrates—can lower cholesterol in other ways, but all these products are used less often than statins.

---

### BASIC SCIENCE AND MEDICAL ADVANCES

Michael S. Brown and Joseph L. Goldstein won the Nobel Prize in 1985 for the discovery of how cells in the body pull cholesterol out of the blood. Dr. George E. Palade, Yale University cell biologist and winner of the 1974 Nobel Prize in Medicine, says of their work: It is "a beautiful example of research that leads from discovery to understanding of biomedical problems at different levels—from that of a given molecule to that of single cells and finally to that of a whole human organism."[38] Their research is also a beautiful example of how the partnership of medicine and basic science can lead to new understanding of heart problems. Brown and Goldstein attribute much of their success to their education and continuing practice as both physicians and lab scientists.

The careers of the prize winners reveal the strong training they received in basic science and medicine. Dr. Brown completed his college degree in chemistry and his medical degree at the University of Pennsylvania. He then served his internship and residency at the Massachusetts General Hospital in Boston and did research at the National Institutes of Health on hereditary disease and the biochemistry of enzyme regulation in the body.[39] Dr. Goldstein attended Washington and Lee University of Virginia for a degree in chemistry and then attended Southwestern Medical School at the University of Texas Health Science Center in Dallas. He did his internship and residency at the Massachusetts General Hospital and trained further in molecular biology at the National Institutes of Health and in medical genetics at the University of Washington.[40] Brown and Goldstein became friends while serving as interns in Boston and researchers at the National Institutes of Health. Sharing both research interests and a passion for duplicate bridge, they later joined one another as professors at the University of Texas Health Science Center. While professors, they not only carried on the biochemistry and molecular biology research that would bring them the Nobel Prize and recognition as worldwide experts on the body's use of cholesterol—they also continued to make rounds as attending physicians at Parkland Memorial Hospital in Dallas.

---

## MINOR SURGERY

If possible, doctors and patients want to avoid major heart surgery such as a heart transplant for congestive heart failure, surgical repair and replacement of heart valves, and coronary artery bypass grafts. Less-invasive surgical procedures that typically involve only a short stay in the hospital and less risk of complications have therefore become increasingly popular.

### Coronary Angioplasty

Along with their use to diagnose heart problems, catheterization procedures can also widen coronary arteries that have become narrow. This procedure is called percutaneous (through the skin) transluminal (inside an artery) coronary angioplasty (blood vessel reshaping), or PTCA.[41] As is done for an angiography, a long tube or catheter is inserted through an artery or vein in the groin area into the heart while doctors view its movement through the veins or arteries on a televised x-ray machine. After a small amount of contrast agent that appears clearly in the x-ray is injected into the coronary arteries and used to identify the location of the blockage, the corrective treatment begins. A smaller catheter that contains a tiny uninflated balloon is pushed inside and through the first tube. When the balloon reaches the blockage in the coronary artery, it is inflated briefly and then deflated. By stretching the artery wall, the inflated balloon will ideally enlarge the diameter of the artery. Another angiography checks to see if the blockage has been removed. Overall, the procedure takes 30 to 90 minutes. (A similar kind of procedure involves guiding a catheter into the heart, positioning it through a narrowed valve, inflating the balloon, and enlarging the opening for blood to flow between chambers.)

More than 90 percent of coronary angioplasties have initial success in clearing the blockage, improving symptoms, and preventing a heart attack. The procedure also proves highly effective in clearing blockages during emergency treatment of persons undergoing a heart attack. The risk of death from coronary angioplasty is less than 1 percent, and the risk of causing a heart attack is less than 3 percent. The procedure can occasionally injure the artery or make the blockage worse. More common than these complications is that about one-third of the blockages return to their original severity in less than one year.

A variation on the procedure involves inserting a stent into the part of the artery that has narrowed after an angioplasty.[42] A stent is a small wire mesh tube inserted into the coronary artery to prop open the narrowed part much like a support prevents a tunnel from collapsing.[43] New developments such as chemically coating the stent with special drugs seem to increase the effectiveness of the device. Although older stents closed up in a month or two in 20 to 40 percent of patients, new stents have been shown to remain open in more than 90 percent of the cases, and even better ones may soon appear on the market.[44]

Still other variations involving heart catheterization sometimes help treat coronary artery disease. Laser ablation uses a tiny laser beam to vaporize plaque along the artery wall, and an atherectomy uses a rotating high-speed cutting drill to shave off plaque.

Compared with major surgery, angioplasty and related procedures are less invasive and expensive, require a shorter recovery for patients, and can be done on patients unable to withstand surgery. Still, they have some limitations. If there are many blockages to correct, if the plaque is calcified or hardened, or if the blockage is at a point the catheter can't get to, the procedures may not be helpful.[45] The ideal patient will have a single well-defined obstruction, good heart function, angina not otherwise controlled by diet or medication, and good general health. That many such patients exist highlights the benefits of these forms of minor surgery.

### Pacemakers

The only effective treatment for a slow heartbeat is a pacemaker.[46] It contains a generator and batteries in a small casing that are connected by wires to the heart. Generating tiny and painless electrical impulses that stimulate the heart, the pacemaker keeps the heartbeat at the appropriate speed and rhythm. The pacemaker's program ideally stimulates the heart based on the person's needs and activity level. It remains passive when the heart beats normally but begins pacing when it senses the heart is beating too slowly. Some pacemakers sense the person's physical activity and accelerate the rate in response to the patient's needs. Technology has improved the capabilities of pacemakers, and implanting the pacemaker is a fairly minor procedure. It takes about one hour and involves staying in the hospital for a day or two.

A variation on such surgery involves the implantation of a cardioverter defibrillator to deal with the life-threatening situation in which the heart begins beating too fast on a recurring basis.[47] These devices are small, about the size of a soap dish, but can monitor the heart rate and give shocks to correct ventricular fibrillation and tachycardia.

## BENEFITS OF IMPROVED TREATMENT FOR HEART DISEASE MORTALITY

### Recent Progress

During the early stages of the decline in heart disease mortality, the period from the mid-1960s to the late 1970s, it appears that changes in lifestyle had more to do with its decline than medical interventions and treatments by physicians. One study focusing on the years from 1968 to 1976 found that medical treatment of clinical ischemic heart disease accounted for 10 percent of the drop, treatment of hypertension for 8.5 percent, and use of coronary care units for 13.5 percent.[48] In contrast, reductions in blood cholesterol levels and cigarette smoking together accounted for 54 percent of the decline. Although both medical interventions and lifestyle appear important, lifestyle had the stronger influence.

Since that time, however, treatments for heart disease have improved dramatically (as have tests to accurately diagnose heart disease at early stages). In contrast, the early progress made in lowering cholesterol and cigarette use has stalled. Treatment of heart disease has therefore become increasingly important in reducing heart disease since the 1970s. This shows in the simple fact that the incidence of heart disease has risen or stayed level, while mortality has declined steadily. Medical treatments of heart disease must account for the pattern.

A study that quantified the contribution of various factors over the period from 1980 to 1990 found that the largest improvement comes from medical treatment.[49] Preventing the occurrence of heart disease through better lifestyles explains about 25 percent of the drop, treatment of these same factors for those with coronary heart disease accounts for about 29 percent of the drop, and treatment of heart disease patients with medical procedures accounts for about 43 percent of the drop. Reducing risk factors among both those with and without coronary heart disease together is important but so is reducing mortality from medical treatment of the disease.

The increasing effectiveness of heart disease treatments is consistent with the rising use of heart disease medications. A study examining trends in the use of heart-related medicines found the following:[50]

- Warfarin use increased from 12 percent in 1990 to 41 percent in 1995 and then to 58 percent in 2002.
- Beta-blocker use increased slowly from 19 percent in 1990 to 20 percent in 1995 and then doubled to 40 percent in 2002.
- Aspirin use increased slowly from 18 percent in 1990 to 19 percent in 1995 and then doubled to 38 percent in 2002.
- Use of ACE inhibitors (including the newer angiotensin receptor blockers) increased from 24 percent in 1990 to 36 percent in 1996 and then to 39 percent in 2002.

The rising use of these medications also shows in a study of heart attack patients in Minneapolis and St. Paul hospitals from 1985 to 1995.[51] Among men, use of beta-blockers rose from 54 to 72 percent, and use of aspirin rose from 26 to 92 percent. Among women, use of beta-blockers rose from 51 to 63 percent, and use of aspirin rose from 20 to 94 percent. High-dose heparin, a blood thinner, rose in use from about 26 percent in 1985 to about 82 percent in 1995. Other medications were used less often as more effective ones became available, but the reliance on improved treatments can account for much of the drop in heart disease mortality among hospital patients.

The use of minor surgical procedures has similarly risen. Across the United States, angioplasty rose from about 2,000 in 1979 to 227,000 in 1988.[52] In the Minneapolis–St. Paul study for the years from 1985 to 1995, angioplasty used for therapeutic purposes rose from about 5 percent to about 34 percent, and thrombolytic therapy rose from about 12 percent to 28 percent.[53]

Other evidence indicates the importance of treatment to the decline in heart disease mortality of those with heart disease. From 1987 to 1994, hospitalization for heart attacks remained stable or increased, but mortality declined, in large part because of improvements in treatments that prevented another heart attack.[54] The improvements, in other words, reflect a shift from fatal to nonfatal heart events.[55] Studies in Sweden, England, New Zealand, and Scotland disclose similar changes.

### Future Progress

The benefits of treatment will likely improve or even accelerate in decades to come. First, the number of statin drugs on the market and the number of users have risen dramatically and will likely continue to rise. Recommendations from research and public health officials call for large increases in the prescription of these drugs. With sales of $15.9 billion in 2000, one estimate is that sales growth will be 12 percent annually over the next several years.[56] Such growth in these products should contribute to advances against heart disease.

Second, many other heart medications, despite their proven benefit, are underused in treating heart disease. The improvements in the use of warfarin, beta-blockers, aspirin, and ACE inhibitors to treat heart disease are remarkable, but according to one study, they still leave room for future advances.[57]

Third, the health of millions has improved from the use of drugs to lower blood pressure. A five- to tenfold increase in the prescription of anti-hypertension drugs occurred from the 1950s through the 1980s, and major reductions in the prevalence of extreme high blood pressure followed.[58] These changes were accompanied by a decline in heart damage related to high blood pressure. However, the downward trend in hypertension has slowed in the 1990s. Renewed efforts to treat hypertension and the harm it brings for heart disease may lead to further benefits in the future.

Still other advances in medication and medical procedures that are now in development may bring even greater benefits in years to come. Although the ideal is to prevent heart disease from occurring, the strategy of identifying those most at risk for heart disease and treating them through medications and minor surgical procedures has done much to contribute to progress against heart disease.

# CHAPTER 5

# Surgical Treatments

On February 24, 1987, 54-year-old Larry King, the host of *Larry King Live* on CNN, had a heart attack.[1] A two- to three-pack-a-day smoker since age 17, he had been told seven years before that he had heart disease, but he had not recognized the seriousness of the problem until a mild pain in his chest sent him to the emergency room at George Washington Hospital in Washington, D.C. In the emergency room, things took a turn for the worse when he felt a terrible aching pain in his right shoulder and right arm. Diagnosing a heart attack, the doctor gave him intravenous fluids with a clot-dissolving drug. Within about five minutes, the medication successfully broke up the clot that blocked the flow of blood to the heart and eliminated the pain. After a stay in the hospital, where he continued to receive clot-dissolving medication and underwent an angioplasty to widen the coronary artery that caused the heart attack, King felt good. Despite tests showing several blockages in his coronary arteries, he rejected the idea of surgery out of hand.

Along with the medication and angioplasty, a change in lifestyle that included losing weight, giving up smoking, and avoiding red meat seemed to keep the symptoms of heart disease away. Four weeks after the heart attack, King returned to his show and to the hard-driving, workaholic life that he enjoyed, and things seemed to be going well. However, in August of that same year, the chest pains started to return, and it became increasingly difficult for him to exert himself. New tests showed that the most serious blockage of the artery had returned and that the risk of another heart attack was high. Despite the change of lifestyle, nonsurgical treatments would likely not work, given a previous lifetime of bad habits and probable genetic predisposition (his father died of a heart attack at age 43). After digesting opinions from two doctors recommending heart bypass surgery, he reluctantly agreed to have the operation.

On December 1, 1987, King underwent the surgery. After opening the chest to access the heart, the surgeons performed a quintuple bypass to deal with blockages. The surgery began at 8:45, ended at 3:05, and appeared to have gone well. Although sore for a few weeks afterward, King found that he experienced less pain than he expected. He soon began seeing visitors, eating, and walking, and after eight days, he was released from the hospital. Tests a year later showed good blood flow and no pain from physical exertion. Fifteen years later and now in his late 60s, King continues to do his show and appears healthy. He needed another angioplasty to reopen a closed artery a few years ago, but he continues to eat a healthy diet, exercise often, and avoid smoking. He can look back and say that the heart attack and bypass surgery profoundly changed his life for the better.

Although a celebrity, Larry King's experience differs little from that of millions of other, less-famous people who have had heart bypass surgery. It seems as if coronary artery bypass surgery has almost become a rite of passage among middle-aged men (less so for women). In 1999, cardiac surgeons performed 571,000 bypass operations in the United States, which makes it the nation's most common type of major surgery. Estimates for the early 1990s suggest that "approximately 1 in every 1000 persons undergoes CABG [coronary artery bypass grafting] on an annual basis, and this procedure results in the expenditures of almost $50 billion annually."[2]

The number of coronary bypass surgeries represents a huge growth in the procedure since its development in 1967. From a level of near zero in that year, the number rose to 180,000 in 1983. The growth has continued since then, reaching 598,000 in 1996 before falling slightly to 571,000 in 1999.[3] Despite the recent drop off (due largely to improvements in alternative techniques such as angioplasty), the numbers more than tripled since 1983.

Other types of open-heart surgery, such as those to replace defective heart valves, correct congenital defects, and transplant healthy hearts into patients with serious heart failure, have increased as well but not nearly as much as bypass surgery. In 1999, coronary bypasses comprised about 76 percent of all open-heart procedures, with the next most common type—valve replacement surgery—comprising only 13 percent (about 96,000). Much less common than either of the other types, heart transplant surgery occurred only 2,184 times.[4] Figure 5.1 depicts the percentages of all open-heart surgeries that involve bypasses, valve replacements, transplants, and all other procedures. The percentage of bypasses far exceeds any other type, indicating that the most important change in the surgical treatment of heart disease comes from bypass surgery.

**Figure 5.1**
**Open-Heart Surgery Procedures (Percentage) in 1999**

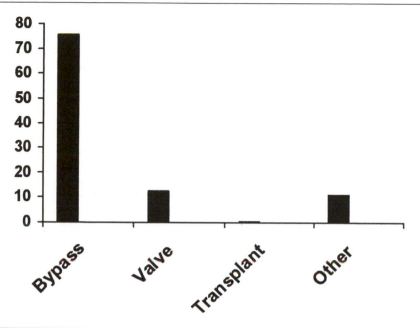

*Source:* American Heart Association, "Open-Heart Surgery Statistics," http:// americanheart.org/presenter.jhtml?identifier = 4674 (accessed October 2002).

It seems, however, that the rise in bypass surgery has been accompanied by controversy over its effectiveness. A highly invasive procedure, bypass surgery not only can produce immediate and long-term complications but may do little more to promote survival than nonsurgical techniques. Success stories like that of Larry King must be balanced by other stories that involve death during the operation, failure of the procedure to open blood flow, recurrence of the blockage a few years after the surgery, and problems of mental capacity resulting from the surgery. Such problems have led to debate over the suitability of the operation and to questions over the contribution of surgical procedures to declining heart disease mortality.

## OPEN-HEART SURGERY

### Heart Bypass

Before presenting the evidence on the effectiveness and value of bypass surgery, it will help to explain the procedure and introduce a few terms.[5]

Coronary artery bypass graft surgery (formally referred to as CABG) represents one surgical form of revascularization or means to restore blood flow (the other form, discussed in the last chapter, is angioplasty, or PTCA). The commonly used shorthand term of heart bypass might misleadingly imply that the procedure involves bypassing the heart, when it in fact involves bypassing blocked parts of the coronary arteries. To avoid misleading terms, while also avoiding acronyms or complex terminology, the discussion to follow refers simply to bypass surgery.

The goal of bypass surgery is to restore the blood supply to the heart muscle by creating new routes, or bypasses, for the blood to flow around blockages in the coronary arteries, much as a bypass road avoids congested areas of a city. The history of the procedure begins with Dr. Alexis Carrel, who developed a technique to stitch small vessels in the early 1900s.[6] His efforts to graft vessels to the heart-blood system in animals were not successful, but Dr. Carrel later won the Nobel Prize in Medicine for this and other innovations in vascular surgery. Efforts in this direction continued on animals, but it was not until the development of a heart-lung machine in the 1950s and 1960s that the bypass procedure became practical for use on humans. In 1967, doctors in Cleveland and Argentina successfully performed coronary bypass surgery and published the results in 1968. The use of the technique then spread quickly.

The key to the procedure is to take vessels from other parts of the body, hook the vessel on one end to a part of the coronary artery just past the blockage and hook the vessel on the other end to the aorta as a source of blood flow. The blood can thus pass through the bypass vessel to the unblocked parts of the coronary artery and feed the heart muscle with oxygen and nutrients. Since alternative routes of blood flow must be constructed for each blockage in the arteries, the grafting process is repeated up to five times as necessary. Surgeons use a vein from the lower leg, an artery from the forearm, or an artery from the inside chest wall to build the new coronary pathway. These vessels are the right size, shape, and length needed for the bypass, but recent research indicates that the arteries better resist new atherosclerosis than a leg vein.

Because precise cutting and sewing actions on coronary arteries are difficult—though not impossible—when the heart continues to beat, most bypass surgery requires a way to circulate blood artificially while the heart is stopped. A pump oxygenator (or heart-lung machine) meets this requirement. It reroutes blood returning from the body into a reservoir that then pumps the blood into an artificial lung. As blood flows through the fine surfaces of the artificial lung or oxygenator, it comes into contact with oxygen gas, absorbs oxygen molecules, and releases carbon dioxide. The blue, unoxygenated blood then becomes red with oxygen and is pumped back into the body through a tube connected to the arterial system. At the same time, refrigeration of the blood cools the body and reduces the need for oxygen, and an anticoagulant (heparin) keeps the blood from clotting as it flows through the oxygenator.

The operation begins with a vertical opening of the skin in the center of the chest, followed by sawing through the breast bone and spreading open the rib cage. After next parting the soft tissue and membrane surrounding the heart, the surgeons free the lower parts of the chest artery to use in the bypass; alternatively, other members of the surgery team harvest a vein or artery to use instead of the chest artery. Before the grafting begins, large doses of the anticoagulant heparin are given to thin the blood, the patient is connected to the heart-lung machine, and the body temperature is lowered by refrigerating the blood as it flows through the heart-lung machine. After the vessels from the heart are clamped, a cold potassium solution is used to make the heart motionless, cold, and relaxed.

The grafting occurs by making an opening into the front wall of the blocked coronary artery and stitching the donor vessel to the opening. The chest artery already has a connection to a source of blood and, if used, does not require grafting on the other end. Otherwise, however, the bypass vessel must be attached to a source of blood. An opening in the wall of the aorta is made and used to connect to the donor vessel. The process is repeated until all major obstructions are bypassed. Then, releasing the clamps allows blood to flow through the artery bypass vessels, and gradually withdrawing the heart-lung system allows the heart to begin beating again. After final checks to make sure all is in order, the surgery ends with closing of the incisions and sending the patient to intensive care for recovery.

Barring postoperative problems, patients can typically leave the hospital about five days after the surgery. They can usually resume most normal activities in about two to three weeks and return to employment and more vigorous activities within four to six weeks. To promote recovery, hospital personnel encourage simple movement right after the surgery and specify a regimen of increasing exercise after leaving the hospital. Stopping smoking, consuming low-fat foods, and implementing a regular exercise program round out the after-surgery goals.

## JOHN H. GIBBON AND THE PUMP OXYGENATOR

At the turn of the twentieth century, doctors vigorously debated the possibility of surgically repairing defects of the heart.[7] Many opposed the idea altogether as reckless and guaranteed to fail. Critics noted that although surgeons could open the chest, they could perform only the simplest of procedures on a beating heart. Stopping the heart for more than a few minutes to allow more complex surgical repairs would kill the patient. Advanced heart surgery would require some way of shutting down or bypassing the heart. Surgeons in 1952 introduced one such method: cooling the body to 30 degrees Celsius (86 degrees Fahrenheit) reduced the need for oxygen enough to stop the heart from beating for a short time. Other efforts to reduce the temperature to 10–20 degrees Celsius (50–68 degrees Fahrenheit) would permit surgeons to stop the heart for up to an hour.[8] However, even this period of time did not allow for complex surgery that heart patients often needed. Another procedure involved circulating blood from the surgery patient through another person but risked harming two rather than one patient.

A more successful solution to the problem, the development of a machine to bypass the heart and lung in circulating blood to the body, came from John H. Gibbon, a professor of surgery at Jefferson Medical College in Philadelphia.[9] After the death of a young patient in 1931, Dr. Gibbon saw the need for a device that would allow the kind of heart surgery his patient needed. He knew the techniques needed to repair heart muscles and valves but lacked the ability to keep the patient alive while stopping the heart. His colleagues dismissed the idea of a machine to bypass and replace the heart and lungs as impossible, but he soon began work on the device. In 1934, he and his wife developed a prototype heart-lung machine or pump oxygenator that he began to test using cats. His first success came in 1935, when he used his machine to keep a cat alive for 26 minutes. He found in the experiments that the machine did not need to replicate the pulsating rhythm of the heart but could pump blood continuously through the artificial lung and the body. However, his work was disrupted by his service in World War II, and the machine remained unused until the 1950s.

With the support of IBM and its engineering division, Gibbon began experimenting after World War II on dogs with his machine. He developed a means of spreading blood over a thin mesh to allow it to absorb oxygen and release carbon dioxide that worked better than previous methods he had used. After finding he could keep dogs alive for more than an hour on the machine, he first used it on a human in 1953.[10] Open-heart surgery on an 18-year-old girl that year proved successful. Continued improvement in the pump oxygenator made it the procedure of choice and made John H. Gibbon a pioneering inventor and heart surgeon.

## Other Surgeries

Open-heart surgery often involves repairing or replacing defective valves that either do not open enough to allow blood into the next chamber or close well enough to prevent blood from flowing or leaking backward into the previous chamber. Like bypass surgery, heart valve surgery requires using a heart-lung machine and stopping the heart. In some cases, surgical repair such as separating parts of the valve that have become fused or adjusting the connection between the valve and the heart muscle can deal with the problem. In other cases, the valve malfunction may be so severe that replacement with a pig valve or artificial valve becomes necessary.

Other types of open-heart surgery repair congenital heart defects, most often in infants and children. For example, procedures can correct problems created by the transposition of the pulmonary and aortic arteries, by the extreme narrowing of the aorta that constricts the flow of blood to the body, by openings in the muscle walls of the heart, and by defective or absent valves. Many such surgeries require use of a heart-lung machine and present serious risks to the patient but also correct life-threatening heart problems.[11]

Heart transplant surgery is less common than the other types of open-heart surgeries. It involves replacing a defective heart with a healthy heart from a recently deceased person.[12] Patients in need of a heart transplant can suffer from a variety of heart problems, including coronary artery disease, cardiomyopathy, congenital heart problems, and valvular heart disease, but all lead to the failure of the heart to pump blood through the body adequately. During the operation, procedures similar to those in bypass surgery are needed to open the chest cavity and attach the patient to a heart-lung machine. The surgeons then remove most of the diseased heart but leave some parts to act as a support for the new heart as it is sewn in place. The new heart can next be positioned and attached to blood vessels.

Heart transplant surgery represents a last resort to dealing with heart disease—one needed for patients who have failed to benefit from all other interventions. At the same time, however, the patients must be otherwise healthy enough to survive major open-heart surgery. Along with the trauma of the surgery, patients face difficulties after surgery because of the tendency of the immune system to reject the new heart tissue, which appears to the body as a foreign substance. To alleviate this problem, medications suppress the immune system, which can make the patient vulnerable to infection and lengthen the period of recovery. If able to manage the difficulties of the surgery and recovery period, patients do well with heart transplants. About 80 percent of patients survive for one year or longer after the procedure, and 50 percent of those receiving heart transplants live nine years or more.

The most serious problem is not finding patients with life-threatening heart failure and the strength to withstand the trauma of the transplant but the lack of donor hearts. While more than two thousand persons received heart transplants in 1999, almost four thousand patients await a donor heart. Well-publicized experiments to install an artificial heart rather than a live heart have so far failed, but continued efforts in this direction could in the future overcome the problem of lack of donor hearts.

## CHRISTIAN BARNARD AND HEART TRANSPLANTS

Over one weekend in 1967, Christian Barnard, a surgeon in Cape Town, South Africa, became the first doctor to transplant a heart into a human being. Recollecting the event, Dr. Barnard said, "On Saturday, I was a surgeon in South Africa, very little known. On Monday, I was world renowned."[13] Indeed, his innovative efforts to find a way to treat patients whose hearts were so damaged that they could not be repaired make him one of the great medical innovators. He never quite expected such renown, recalling, "I did not even inform the hospital superintendent of what we were doing." Still, the idea of giving one person the heart of another sparked worldwide interest and led to unprecedented publicity for a surgeon. He later became a global celebrity known for his eccentric lifestyle along with his medical achievements.

The son of a poor preacher in South Africa, Barnard became a family physician but then studied cardiac surgery in the United States. Returning to South Africa, he began experimenting with heart surgery in animals and performed kidney transplants on humans. In 1967, Barnard led a 30-man medical team in transplanting the heart of a 25-year-old woman killed in a motor vehicle accident into a 55-year-old man with a damaged heart. The heart recipient lived only 18 days and died of pneumonia, a result of the suppression of his immune system to prevent rejection of the foreign tissue of the new heart. It would take many years before drugs could successfully deal with the problem of rejection, but Barnard had spearheaded a significant medical advance that would save thousands of lives in decades to come.

Young and handsome, Barnard became an international celebrity who spent "as much time in nightclubs as operating theatres."[14] Dating beautiful actresses and traveling across the world to promote his work, he became the subject of newspaper articles and gossip columns as well as the object of controversy in medical circles for his work as a surgeon and his promotion of cosmetics. He later attempted to use the heart of a monkey to keep a desperately ill patient alive, tried to find a way to slow the aging process, and supported euthanasia for terminally ill patients. His healthy ego offended many but also gave him the courage to push the boundaries of medical science. He died at age 78 in 2001 while vacationing in Cyprus.

## THE CASE FOR BYPASS SURGERY

### Benefits

Bypass surgery, the most common open-heart procedure, has generated the most debate over its benefits and overuse. According to the American Heart Association, the main purpose of bypass surgery is to relieve the symptoms of angina and ischemia. The condition recognized as suitable for bypass surgery is moderate to severe angina that does not respond to medications. In addition, the procedure is increasingly used in cases where the symptoms of angina are mild to moderate but where there are indications of serious underlying heart conditions that threaten the life of the patient.

Given the goal to relieve angina, the bypass operation appears to work well, with about 90 percent of patients experiencing less pain from angina, greater ability to exercise, and less need for anti-angina medicine. About 70 percent of bypass patients fully recover and resume normal activities, and about 20 percent gain partial relief, but for 5 to 10 percent, the bypass collapses within a year.[15] Examining longer-term effects, one textbook summarizes the findings of the outcomes of bypass surgery: "After 5 years, approximately three fourths of surgically treated patients can be predicted to be free from an ischemic event, sudden death, occurrence of myocardial infarction, or return of angina; about half remain free for approximately 10 years, and about 15 percent for 15 or more years."[16]

Rather than describing the progress of bypass patients, better measures of the effectiveness of bypass surgery for relieving pain come from comparing surgically and medically treated patients with angina. In one comparative study, 62 percent of the surgery group were free of chest pain after five years, while 29 percent of the medical group were free of chest pain.[17] However, these benefits appear to diminish after five years. Thus, for some patients with persistent angina that does not respond to medical methods and other less-invasive procedures, bypass surgery does well in relieving symptoms.

The effects of bypass surgery on survival rather than pain relief are less clear and harder to demonstrate. On the surface, the outcome statistics look pretty good. After 10 years, about 80 percent of the bypass patients have survived; given the precarious cardiac health of those that undergo the procedure and their high risk of a heart attack, such a survival rate makes the surgery appear successful. However, if similar patients who do not undergo the surgery have an equally high survival rate, these figures can be misleading. As with evaluation of the benefits of bypass surgery for pain relief, evaluating the benefits of bypass surgery requires comparisons with patients who are treated with medications, nonsurgical procedures, and lifestyle changes. The key to making such comparisons is the random assignment of subjects to the surgical and medical treatments. This ensures that the two groups do not differ in the seriousness of the underlying disease and the risks of death. Three major studies using randomized trials and done during the 1970s provide information on the survival benefits of bypass surgery.[18]

The first study of Veterans Administration patients found no significant differences in the 11-year survival of patients assigned to the two groups and thus overall indicates no survival benefits from heart bypass procedures. However, more refined analysis suggests that the highest-risk subsets of patients did experience a survival benefit. In a second study, funded by the National Institutes of Health, no survival differences appeared between the surgery and medication groups overall, but some benefit of surgery came to those at higher risk. A third study in Europe found significant improvement only among those with more serious heart disease in three vessels. For those with the most serious disease, 91 percent of the surgical group survived over the first eight years compared with 73 percent of the nonsurgical group. No survival differences appeared among groups with less-serious disease in one or two vessels.

## Recent Improvements

These studies may in some ways underestimate the benefits of the procedure. The trials occurred before two innovations that have improved the effectiveness of the surgery became common—using the chest (internal mammary) artery in the surgery rather than using the leg vein, and using aspirin after the surgery to improve blood flow. Whereas 40 to 60 percent of bypasses using the leg veins remain unblocked after 10 to 12 years, 90 percent of bypasses using the chest artery remain unblocked.[19] Similarly, the use of aspirin after bypass surgery significantly improves the survival rate.[20] The more common use of the chest artery and aspirin these days likely would increase the survival rate of surgical patients relative to medically treated patients.

Early studies generally excluded high-risk patients because surgeons thought during the early years of the procedure that such patients were not suited for the difficult operation. Based on evidence that has accumulated since the 1970s, it now appears that high-risk patients benefit most from bypass surgery. In fact, recent decades have seen bypasses done for increasingly older and increasingly more serious forms of heart disease. Including the high-risk patients who benefit most from bypass surgery in randomized trials would certainly reveal an increase in the rate of survival advantage of those undergoing bypass surgeries.

Improvements of techniques and training of surgeons since the 1970s, a period in which the operation remained new, also have done much to improve the risks of the surgery. Deaths during the surgery now occur in only about 3 percent of patients, and yearly reports show a steady decline in deaths from bypass surgery through the 1990s.[21] The downward trend seems all the more positive when noting that the patients having the surgery are increasingly older and less healthy. A study of patient records gathered by the Society of Thoracic Surgeons found that bypass patients in the 1990s were "significantly older, sicker and have a higher risk than a decade ago."[22] Even so, bypass mortality rates have declined substantially, and these trends "highlight the excellent progress in the care of CABG patients achieved during the past decade."[23]

Improvements in technique may have benefited women even more than men. Early studies indicated that the operative mortality for women having bypass surgery reached 5 percent. However, a recent study sponsored by the National Institutes of Health that enrolled 1,829 subjects reported in 1998 that survival rates are equally high for men and women.[24] Improvements in techniques mean that it is just as safe for women as men.

### Eligibility

The eligibility criteria for bypass surgery follow from the findings of the randomized trials.[25] Since surgery provided low-risk patients no added survival gain beyond medical treatment, but did extend the life of high-risk patients, the recommendations limit bypass surgery to patients with quite specific and serious conditions.

First, among patients without severe angina symptoms, bypass surgery is warranted for those with a blockage in the left main coronary artery, severe blockages in three or more coronary arteries, and severely impaired function of the heart's main pumping chamber. Second, for those with severe angina, bypass surgery is warranted to relieve the pain but brings little in the way of survival benefit.

Even under these conditions, bypass surgery works best in combination with other treatments. Efforts to deal with atherosclerosis should begin with medications and angioplasty, and bypass should be used after these approaches fail. The need to hold bypass surgery in reserve is particularly important for younger heart patients. Because bypass vessels have a life of about 15 years, and second bypass surgeries are generally less successful than the first, surgery on younger patients will likely create treatment problems later in life. After one bypass, it may be necessary to limit treatment to medication and angioplasty.

Physicians also view changes in lifestyles as a crucial part of bypass surgery. Many may have once seen bypass surgery as a cure for heart disease, one that allowed patients to return to unhealthy smoking, eating, and exercising habits. Today, we know that the underlying problems that cause the heart disease must also be addressed if the heart problems are not to return soon after the surgery. Bypass surgery remains just one component of the overall treatment of the heart patient.

## THE CASE AGAINST BYPASS SURGERY

### Overuse

In reviewing the randomized studies, more extreme critics of bypass surgery assert that no evidence demonstrates the survival benefits of the procedure. However, most physicians, even those critical of the routine use of bypass surgery, recognize the benefits of the procedure for those who fall into the high-risk category. Their concern comes from what appears to be the overuse of the procedure for patients who do not meet the strict criteria for the effective use of the procedure. The number of bypass surgeries rose steadily from the time of the studies demonstrating only limited effectiveness of the procedure in the 1970s to the peak in the mid-1990s. Since then, the peak has dropped only slightly.

Can all these surgeries be justified as contributing to the survival of heart patients or the relief of severe symptoms? Is bypass surgery being used as a last resort after other treatments have been given time to work? Critics say no and cite a variety of evidence in their favor.

Studies evaluating the decision to use bypass surgery find that errors are commonly made. For example, one 1988 study in the *Journal of the American Medical Association* had a nine-member panel review the records of bypass surgery patients. The panel found that 56 percent of the surgeries were appropriate, 30 percent were performed for equivocal reasons, and 14 percent for inappropriate reasons.[26] Assuming that those performed for equivocal reasons could have best been delayed suggests that 44 percent of the bypass surgeries may have been unnecessary. With 571,000 bypasses in 1999, the 44 percent figure translates into more than 250,000 possibly unneeded surgeries in one year alone.

In addition, studies comparing the United States with other high-income nations have found excess use of bypass surgery. One study published in *The New England Journal of Medicine* compared two groups who had heart attacks in 1991: Medicare beneficiaries in the United States and elderly patients in Ontario, Canada. The study found that 10.6 percent of the American patients underwent heart bypass surgery compared with 1.4 percent of the Canadian patients. Yet, the one-year mortality rates for the patients were identical. In conclusion, the authors state, "The strikingly higher rates of use of cardiac procedures in the United States, as compared with Canada, do not appear to result in better long-term survival rates for elderly U.S. patients with acute myocardial infarction."[27]

Comparisons with Canada, where the diagnosis of heart disease and the population of patients may differ, could artificially exaggerate the use of bypass surgery in the United States. However, comparisons with many other high-income nations indicate much the same. Although most European nations show lower rates of heart bypass surgery, they have in many cases similar or lower mortality rates from heart disease and longer life expectancy than the United States.

Given these country differences, it appears that in the United States, "patients and doctors often don't give medication and lifestyle changes a chance" before resorting to surgery.[28] It takes longer to see the gains from medical treatment than from surgery. However, while the gains from surgery are immediate, they decrease over time; while the gains from medical and lifestyle treatment take longer to emerge, they can last a lifetime. In other words, bypass surgery does not cure the underlying cause and afterward requires medication and lifestyle change anyway. So, why not skip the bypass surgery and go right to the medication and lifestyle change?

A less-generous explanation of the high rates of bypass surgery in the United States focuses on the funding for the health care system. The fee-for-service health care system, in contrast to the single-payer systems of most European nations, brings prestige and financial rewards to hospitals and physicians who perform expensive surgeries.[29] Some more extreme critics call bypass surgery a procedure that does more to enrich doctors and hospitals than improve health. Although certainly excessive, such claims highlight the incentives for use of surgery over less-invasive procedures.

## Dangers

Even if bypass surgery had demonstrated better long-term survival benefits, critics wonder if the benefits would outweigh several risks to health that bypass surgery creates. First, bypass surgery may actually promote heart disease. Because injuries to artery walls promote the accumulation of plaque, and grafting of vessels creates wounds in the coronary arteries, it follows that bypass surgery can promote the process of plaque buildup and lead to the rapid closure of the bypass. Thus, 5 to 10 percent of the bypasses fail within one year, and by 10 years, 40 percent of vein grafts are severely obstructed and require more treatment or another bypass.[30] Grafts using arteries, which are designed to carry blood at a higher pressure than veins, fail less often than grafts using veins but do not last indefinitely. By 15 years, the usual life of a bypass, most grafts have become obstructed and require new surgery or other kinds of treatment.

Second, the likelihood of death during surgery, although usually no more than 3 percent,[31] still means that there are thousands of deaths each year from bypass surgery. The risks of death from surgery must be balanced by the risks of death from going without surgery, but if the survival benefits of surgery are modest, patients might decide not to put themselves through an operation that claims the lives of about three of one hundred cases.

Third, bypass surgery and other surgeries that use a heart-lung machine to replace a beating heart may produce brain problems. Roughly 1.5 to 5.2 percent of bypass surgeries result in a stroke and likely brain problems.[32] Clamping the aorta during the surgery can knock tiny clumps of plaque into the blood stream that cause a stroke by lodging in narrow passageways in the brain. Among those who come through the surgery without brain damage, many will suffer from longer-term decline in their cognitive abilities. In one study from Duke University, researchers found

that 42 percent of patients who underwent bypass surgery showed significant decline on tests of mental ability five years later.[33] The long-term
harm may result from the spread of fatty particles after clamping of the
aorta and from the inability of the heart-lung machine to pump blood to
the brain as effectively as the heart. After still more years, bypass surgery
can increase the risk of dementia, although the evidence for this result is
less strong than that for the other forms of cognitive decline.[34]

Fourth, perhaps less serious and long-lasting than brain damage but
still worrisome, is the emergence of depression after bypass surgery. Estimates suggest that from one-third to three-quarters of bypass patients,
particularly those at older ages, face mental fatigue and overwhelming
sadness after the surgery.[35] For most, the problem resolves itself within
six months but nonetheless brings serious psychological pain to postoperative patients. The depression may stem from temporary alterations of
the brain chemistry brought on by anesthesia or hypothermia, or from the
stress and worry about the procedure. In any case, the problem represents
a side effect of the surgery that might, just like physical recovery, require
more treatment.

## CORONARY BYPASS SURGERY AND DECLINING
## HEART DISEASE MORTALITY

The debates over the advantages and disadvantages of bypass surgery
make it difficult to determine the contribution it has made to declining
heart disease mortality. It is clear that the growth of such surgery, which
began to spread around 1970, has coincided with the steady decline of
heart disease since the late 1960s. Perhaps the coinciding trends indicate
that bypass surgery has saved and extended a sufficiently large number
of lives to contribute to the declining mortality rates. In fact, such a contribution appears to be modest, although perhaps increasing over time.

In an examination of the downward trend in heart disease mortality
between 1968 and 1976, one study made calculations to show that coronary bypass surgery accounted for only 3.5 percent of the decline.[36] The
study notes that the surgery may have increased the quality of life of the
patients but finds little evidence that it did much to extend their lives. In
reviewing trends for much the same period, another study concludes,
"While the contribution of CABG surgery to an improved prognosis in
patients with coronary heart disease is real and certainly important for
the individual fortunate enough to be in the good-risk post surgical group,
the impact on cardiovascular morality and total mortality in the United
States is small."[37]

In more recent years, the benefits may have improved. Since bypass
surgery has been used more since the 1970s to help high-risk patients,
those most likely to die without the procedure, the gains in longevity may

have increased as well. A more recent study of the years from 1980 to 1990 used a simulation model and determined that the major cause of the decline in coronary heart disease came from medical and surgical treatments of the disease.[38] Treatments such as the use of clot-dissolving drugs and procedures such as angioplasty and bypass surgery explain about 43 percent of the drop in deaths from coronary artery disease during the period. These results thus show a stronger effect of the treatment of heart disease for survival than did studies of earlier decades.

The study did not aim to separate the individual effects of the various treatments, which makes it hard to isolate the particular benefits of bypass surgery. However, the model assumes that among those with coronary heart disease, the probability of experiencing a heart attack is 10 percent lower for those having had bypass surgery than those not having had it. Combining this benefit with the 8 percent growth in bypass operations during the 10 years suggests that bypass surgery contributed to the improvement in heart disease mortality.

Surgical treatments other than bypass operations likely have done little to add to these treatment benefits. The replacement of defective valves, the corrections of congenital heart abnormalities, and the transplantation of failing and healthy hearts have extended the lives of many. However, relative to the use of bypass surgery to correct coronary heart disease, the small numbers of these other operations mean they can contribute less to the decline in mortality rates from heart disease.

New techniques of bypass surgery may in the future do more to produce survival benefits. Performance of the surgery without the heart-lung machine—"off pump" in common terminology—may limit the dangers and increase the benefits of the surgery. This minimally invasive bypass surgery involves making a small incision between the ribs that allows the surgeon to view the heart with special optical equipment. The procedure is then done by viewing the heart on a monitor rather than with direct sight and by passing surgical instruments through the viewing tube or another small incision. The surgery is performed on the beating heart but relies on a platform or stabilizer that makes the part of the heart being operated on relatively immobile.[39] A computer helps the surgeon manipulate the surgical instruments.

Although it requires expensive equipment, complex surgical techniques, and special surgical skills, minimally invasive bypass surgery reduces the incidence of stroke, the need for blood transfusions, and the risks of operative mortality.[40] The costs to the patient in terms of money, side effects, and length of hospital stay are also lessened. By not using the heart-lung machine, problems of depression and loss of cognitive skills can be avoided. Moreover, the technique can be used on fragile patients who could not undergo the more invasive bypass surgery.

So far the technique has been limited to single-bypass grafts in the coronary artery that is in the front of the heart and easily accessible through the tiny incisions, but further advances in technology may make it possible to work on other parts of the heart. In the meantime, the American Heart Association Council on Cardio-Thoracic and Vascular Surgery suggests that the procedures sound promising but need more study: "Neither [type of minimally invasive bypass] procedure can be given an unqualified endorsement until more data on their effectiveness is obtained and analyzed."[41]

Continued research on and improvements in the technique could mean that surgical methods will contribute more to declining heart disease in the future than they have in the past. Based on the evidence we have over the past decades, it appears that surgical procedures made only small contributions to the progress against heart disease early on and have done somewhat more to save lives in recent decades.

# PART III

# Lifestyle

# CHAPTER 6

# Tobacco Use

Early users of tobacco in Europe made grandiose claims about its powers to cure bodily ills and stimulate the brain. For example, Jean Nicot declared in the late sixteenth century that rubbing a tobacco ointment on the body would eliminate tumors, which led French royalty to take tobacco in the form of snuff as a preventive measure (Nicot's promotion of tobacco led biologists to name the tobacco plant genus *Nicotiana*, after him). Walter Raleigh, who did much to encourage the spread of tobacco in England during the late sixteenth and early seventeenth centuries, associated smoking with adventure, virility, and style. In describing the tobacco craze in England that Raleigh would help inspire, observers commented that smokers "declare also that their brain is lulled by a pleasing drunkenness."[1]

Despite such claims, many realized early on that tobacco could harm one's health. King James I of England wrote in 1604 that tobacco is a "custom loathsome to the eye, hateful to the nose, harmful to the brain, dangerous to the lungs."[2] The link between smoking and diseases of the lungs would seem obvious, as most anyone could understand that inhaling smoke might leave harmful residue in lung tissue. However, some came to recognize a less-obvious link between heart disease and smoking. An 1848 book on clinical medicine suggested that tobacco caused impairment of the heart, an 1862 book mentioned cigarettes as a cause of angina, an 1889 book used the term "tobacco angina" to describe the heart problems of smokers, and an 1893 report concluded from a postmortem examination that smoking had been responsible for contraction of the walls of the blood vessels, including the arteries of the heart.[3]

In 1912, Dr. Herbert H. Tidswell authored a book on the harm of tobacco that contained several stories about smoking and heart problems. He reported that one patient suffered from "cardiac irregularity [as] a frequent consequence of tobacco smoking [and] never suffers from any cardiac disorder, unless exposed to tobacco fumes."[4] As a result, the man "dare not sit in the smoking room of his club, or in the smoking compartment of a railroad carriage." Another story related by an American doctor illustrates the addictiveness as well as the harm to the heart of tobacco:

[The doctor] was consulted one day by a clergyman, aged fifty; he confessed he had been a great smoker, and for the last month his mind had been greatly impressed with his sin and shame, and he sought to abandon it. He determined to enter his church on Sunday free from his usual indulgence. On rising to open the Church Service he found himself blind and unable to articulate. He almost fell down; he was taken home; when his doctor arrived the patient said, "you need not be troubled, just hand me my tobacco box and I shall be well in two minutes, this is simply a reaction of my nervous system, consequent upon abstinence from my usual indulgence"; he took a chew and slowly recovered. A few weeks later he died from heart disease.[5]

These and many other stories convinced Tidwell of the heart risks created by tobacco use.

Studies some half a century later did indeed confirm early suspicions. The emerging evidence was first summarized systematically in 1964 by a report from the surgeon general on smoking.[6] The report concluded that cigarette smoking was a major independent risk factor for heart attack and sudden cardiac death. This evidence certainly concerned smokers but had an encouraging implication as well: smoking-caused heart disease could be prevented without surgery, medications, or weight loss—it simply required smokers to give up the habit and nonsmokers to never start. Control of smoking had much promise for reducing heart disease, and the 1964 report of the surgeon general marks the start of large-scale public health efforts to lessen cigarette and tobacco use. The early publicity on this topic did indeed reduce both smoking and heart disease, but more recently, the progress against smoking has slowed.

## HARM OF TOBACCO USE

### Cigarettes

If the anecdotes of Tidswell and others fall short of scientific standards of proof, they nonetheless prove consistent with modern statistical studies. Consider some of the facts regarding cigarette smoking and heart disease.[7] For males over age 35, deaths from coronary heart disease are

1.9 times (or 90 percent) higher among smokers than "never smokers" and 1.4 times higher for former smokers than never smokers; for females the same ages, deaths are 1.8 times higher for smokers and 1.3 times higher for former smokers than never smokers. For those age 35–64, when risks of death are otherwise low, male smokers have heart disease mortality rates 2.8 times higher than never smokers, and female smokers have rates 3.0 times higher than never smokers.

A British study of more than 34,000 male doctors over a 40-year period from 1951 to 1991 further confirms the special risks faced by cigarette smokers.[8] The study has two advantages. First, by examining the effects of smoking among an affluent and highly educated group of men, it eliminates the possibility that economic deprivation and low education, rather than smoking, cause heart problems. Second, it followed the sample for a period of 40 years, a period long enough for about 20,000 of the sample to have died and for researchers to examine the long-term effect of smoking. For coronary heart disease, the mortality rates for former smokers were 1.19 times higher than for nonsmokers, and the rates for current smokers were 1.56 times higher than for nonsmokers. In addition, the degree of smoking proved important. Relative to never smokers, coronary heart disease death rates were 1.4 times higher for light smokers (1–14 cigarettes per day), 1.56 times higher for moderate smokers (15–24 cigarettes per day), and 1.79 times higher for heavy smokers (25 or more cigarettes per day).

These relative risks of death translate into perhaps more meaningful numbers. At ages under 65, cigarette use accounts for about 45 percent of male deaths from coronary artery disease and about 41 percent of female deaths from coronary artery disease. The percentages fall for ages over 65, when risks of nonsmoking disease increase, but the percentages of smoking-related heart disease deaths still equal 21 percent for men and 12 percent for women.[9] Due to the early death from coronary heart disease, smoking caused 514,026 years of potential life lost for men and 185,580 for women over the five years from 1995 to 1999.[10] These deaths make heart disease the largest source of smoking-related deaths, even greater than lung cancer. Combining all smoking-caused deaths further indicates the harm of the habit. Smokers on average live 6.5 years less than nonsmokers, and each cigarette costs 11 minutes of life.[11]

Worse, the harm of smoking for heart disease is synergistic.[12] That is, cigarette smoking not only brings harm in its own right but also amplifies the harm of other risk factors. Hypertension, high cholesterol, and diabetes do more to cause severe heart disease when combined with smoking. Moreover, smoking impairs the effectiveness of drugs used to treat heart disease. For women, smoking combined with birth control pills increases coronary heart disease.[13]

Low-yield cigarettes with reduced tar, nicotine, harmful chemicals, and additives bring little benefit in reducing the risks of cigarettes for coronary heart disease. Tar content—the particles contained in the residue or by-product of the burning of tobacco that are inhaled with tobacco smoke—is a major source of the harmful effects of tobacco use on health (but also a major source of tobacco flavor). Use of low-tar cigarettes would therefore seem to bring health gains. Similarly, reducing the amounts of nicotine and other harmful products in cigarette tobacco would also seem advantageous. However, the evidence on the benefits of low-tar and low-nicotine cigarettes for heart disease appears mixed.[14] Smokers of these products often use more cigarettes, puff more often, or inhale more strenuously to get the same amount of nicotine and therefore the same amount of tar, chemicals, and additives as in regular cigarettes. Even if safer cigarettes actually brought the expected health gains, many experts hesitate to recommend them. They worry that a switch to such products may reduce the likelihood of stopping altogether—the best way to eliminate the harm of tobacco. Sadly, the greater use of low-tar cigarettes over the decades has done little to reduce the disease burden of smoking.

### Other Tobacco Products

Heart disease comes from cigar use as well as cigarette use. In one study, men who smoked cigars (but not cigarettes or pipes) had a risk for cardiovascular disease 27 percent higher than that for men who smoked no tobacco product.[15] Moreover, the risks rose with the number of cigars smoked: those who smoked less than five cigars a day had a risk 20 percent higher, while those who smoked five or more had a risk 56 percent higher. The harm of cigar use does not reach that for cigarette use because cigar smokers seldom inhale fumes directly into their lungs as cigarette smokers do. However, even if not inhaled intentionally, cigar smokers breathe in smoke from the air and absorb harmful chemicals through the mouth, both of which increase the chance of developing heart disease.

Smokeless tobacco also contributes to heart disease, although it does so in less-apparent ways than cigar and cigarette smoking. Even more so than from use of cigars, use of smokeless tobacco involves the absorption of harmful chemicals through the mouth cavity. As a result, smokeless tobacco can, according to one study, raise the risk of cardiovascular deaths by 40 percent (compared with 90 percent for those who smoked 15 or more cigarettes a day).[16] Although less severe than smoking cigarettes, the harm of smokeless tobacco for heart disease is real and serious.

One other product of tobacco use injures nonsmokers as well as smokers. Environmental tobacco smoke, or secondhand smoke, comes from the burning of a cigarette or cigar and the smoke exhaled by a smoker. Nonsmokers sharing space inside buildings, homes, and motor vehicles with smokers inhale environmental tobacco smoke (called passive or involuntary smoking). Although research on the harm of passive smoking has created much controversy, figures suggest that long-term exposure to secondhand smoke increases the risk of death by about 30 percent and results in 35,000–62,000 premature deaths a year.[17] For example, nonsmokers living with smoking spouses experience an average increase of 25 percent in the risks of coronary heart disease.[18] The exposure to secondhand smoke affects workers as well as spouses. In one 10-year study of female nurses, subjects exposed to environmental tobacco smoke at work increased their risk of heart disease by 58 percent, and subjects exposed to environmental tobacco smoke at home increased their risks by 91 percent.[19]

In addition to its long-term harm, passive smoking may bring short-term harm. After a 30-minute exposure to environmental tobacco smoke, nonsmokers experience a substantial reduction in the coronary circulation of blood.[20] The results suggest that even a little secondhand smoke is dangerous.[21] If exposure to secondhand smoke for just 30 minutes affects the heart, then it justifies the need for smoke-free workplaces, restaurants, and bars. Indeed, a study of bartenders in San Francisco before and after a smoking ban in bars revealed rapid improvement in their respiratory health with the ban.[22]

Criticisms of studies of passive smoking remain.[23] Effects of small doses of secondhand smoke are difficult to detect, particularly in comparison to the effects of active smoking, and studies often reach different conclusions. The scientific evidence about environmental tobacco smoke is not nearly as overwhelming as it is for cigarette use.[24] Still, the potential for damage given the exposure of large numbers of nonsmokers to the tobacco smoke of others makes it an important public health issue.

## CELEBRITY SMOKERS AND HEART ATTACKS

The list of celebrity smokers who have died from cancer is long and well known: film actor Humphrey Bogart, composer Leonard Bernstein, singer Nat "King" Cole, entertainer Sammy Davis, Jr., corporate founder and animator Walt Disney, television actor Michael Landon, newsman Edward R. Murrow, baseball player Babe Ruth, television producer Ed Sullivan, and film actor John Wayne. Perhaps less well known are celebrity smokers who have died or suffered from heart problems. For example, Lucille Ball, the comedian starring in I Love Lucy, The Lucy Show, and Here's Lucy on television from 1951 to 1974, smoked heavily until her death in 1989 at age 77. President Lyndon Baines Johnson smoked two to three packs of cigarettes a day until his first heart attack in 1955. After serving as vice president and president, he resumed the habit in 1971, suffered another heart attack in 1972, and died of a heart attack in 1973. Other cigarette smokers who have survived heart attacks (such as broadcaster Larry King and public television newsman Jim Lehrer) have improved their survival chances by quitting, but loss of life from smoking-caused heart disease among celebrities and others remains a serious problem.[25]

## HOW DOES TOBACCO USE DAMAGE THE HEART?

The connection between tobacco use and heart disease may be less obvious than the connection between smoking and lung problems, but it is just as real. In simple terms, the chemicals found in cigarettes—ammonia (in harsh cleansers), arsenic (in rat poison), cyanide (in rat poison), hydrogen cyanide (in gas-chamber poison), methanol (in rubbing alcohol), methane (in rocket fuel), butane (in lighter fluid), formaldehyde (in preservation of body tissue), and cadmium (in batteries)—would seem to harm all parts of the body.[26] In addition, however, scientists have identified numerous mechanisms that link smoking to heart damage.[27]

### Atherosclerosis

Narrowing of the coronary arteries by the accumulation of plaque develops over a long time period but may begin when the chemicals in tobacco smoke damage the lining of the vessel walls. Normally, a thin Teflon-like layer of cells that coat the lining of healthy blood vessels ensures smooth blood flow. However, chemicals in tobacco smoke can damage the walls. The damage causes inflammation, attracts immune cells and blood clots, and allows fats and plaque to stick to the area. The accumulation of these materials in the coronary arteries has the consequence of restricting the flow of blood to the heart. In addition, the nicotine in tobacco products leads to the release of epinephrine and norepinephrine, which then cause the release of stored fats into the bloodstream. The released fats allow smokers and tobacco users to skip meals but also can stick to the vessel walls. Compared with nonsmokers, smokers tend to have lower levels of HDL blood cholesterol, the good cholesterol that removes harmful lipids from the blood. For example, a three-year study of more than 10,000 subjects found that current cigarette smoking led to a 50 percent increase in the progress of atherosclerosis, past smoking to a 25 percent increase, and environmental tobacco smoke to a 20 percent increase.[28]

### Vessel Constriction

Along with contributing to the narrowing of arteries with plaque, smoking and tobacco use can obstruct the flow of blood to the heart in another way. They constrict the vessels by reducing the production of chemicals that dilate the arteries (such as prostacyclin) and by reducing the activity of a substance in the blood that instructs the blood vessels to expand (nitrous oxide). Blood vessels of smokers do not, as a result, respond as well as those of nonsmokers to the demand for more blood during physical exertion. When the heart beats fast, the coronary arteries need to widen or dilate to increase the flow of oxygen-rich blood to the heart muscle. That they do not dilate as well for smokers as for nonsmokers (or for users of snuff and chew as for nonusers) limits the ability of smokers (and other tobacco users) to strengthen their hearts through exercise. And for those with existing heart disease, vessel constriction increases angina pain.

### Thrombosis

Smokers have elevated levels of a blood protein called fibrinogen and small blood cells called platelets that play a central role in thrombosis or blood-clot formation. Fibrinogen and platelets contribute to the buildup of plaque and, more seriously, may lead to large blood clots in the vessels. If clots block the flow of blood through the coronary arteries, they can cause a heart attack. In other words, smoking alters the clotting mechanism of the blood in ways that increase the risks of thrombosis and damage to the heart.

### Increased Oxygen Demand

By raising blood pressure and heart rate, smoking and other forms of tobacco use increase the demand of the heart for oxygen by about 10 percent. Nicotine from cigarettes is quickly delivered to the body through the lungs, produces a rush of epinephrine and norepinephrine, and provides a pleasant shot of energy. The adrenaline speeds the heartbeat, makes the arteries squeeze tight, raises blood pressure slightly, and puts more strain on the heart. Experiments show that smoking raises blood pressure by about 25 mm Hg within only five minutes. These physical changes also occur with the use of cigars and smokeless tobaccos, which allow the body to absorb nicotine through the lining of the mouth rather than the linings of the lungs (smoking cessation aids containing nicotine can have the same effect). Whatever the source of the nicotine, the added strain it places on the heart and vessels contributes to the steady development of heart disease.

### Reduced Oxygen Delivery

At the same time it increases the demand of the heart for oxygen, smoking reduces the capacity of the blood to carry oxygen. The reduction comes from the absorption by the blood of carbon monoxide contained in cigarette smoke. Red blood cells and hemoglobin (which carries oxygen in red blood cells) are quicker to bind with the carbon monoxide than with oxygen. Because carbon monoxide replaces needed oxygen, it is poisonous in large doses (and a recognized means of committing suicide when breathed from automobile exhaust). In small doses, it still does damage by reducing the oxygen available to the heart as well as to other parts of the body. It can also contribute to an irregular heartbeat and raise the risk of sudden cardiac arrest.

## BENEFITS OF QUITTING TOBACCO USE

### Reducing Health Risks

More so than for lung cancer, the ill effects of smoking on the heart immediately begin to reverse upon stopping the habit. The risk of death from heart disease falls by 50 percent within one year of quitting and then continues to fall more gradually.[29] Within 15 years, the risks of former smokers and never smokers no longer differ. The short-term gains come from reduced tendencies for blood clots to form in the vessels, and the long-term gains come from improved functioning of the coronary arteries. These benefits of quitting occur among women as well as men, among older persons as well as younger persons, and among heavy smokers as well as light smokers. On average, then, smoking cessation increases life expectancy by 2.3 years for men and 2.8 years for women, but those who stop at younger ages enjoy even more years of added life.[30]

Stopping smoking brings special benefits to those who have already survived a heart attack. Within three years after the heart attack, those victims who stopped smoking have risks of a recurrence that differ little from victims who never smoked and have substantially lower risks than those who continue to smoke.[31] It is never too late to profit from a smoke-free lifestyle.

California has provided a real-life experiment that illustrates the improvements in health realized by lower smoking. A large, aggressive antitobacco program implemented in the state in 1989 not only accelerated the decline in the rate of cigarette consumption but also was associated with lower rates of heart disease.[32] According to one estimate, the program led to 33,300 fewer deaths from heart disease in California between 1989 and 1997. Cutbacks in the program ultimately reduced its effectiveness, but the early success indicates the potential for population health to improve from changes in smoking behavior. A more recent ban of smoking in Helena, Montana, seems to have had even more striking effects on heart attacks (see the related story in the box).

Along with extending life, smoking cessation makes daily living more enjoyable in many ways. Since the breathing and heart problems of smokers restrict their activities, former smokers can take newfound pleasure in physical activity, sexual relationships, and feelings of healthfulness. Compared with continuing smokers, former smokers save money once paid for cigarettes and spend less time and money visiting doctors and being hospitalized. Nonsmokers (including fetuses, infants, and young children who are particularly vulnerable to smoking by parents) also benefit from reduced smoking by being better able to avoid secondhand smoke and enjoy clean air. Nonsmokers may also enjoy economic gains from a decrease in smoking prevalence among adults. The change results in fewer hospitalizations for heart attacks, lower medical costs, and diminished spending for public medical insurance programs.[33]

---

### IMMEDIATE BENEFITS OF A SMOKING BAN

Dr. Robert Shepard and Dr. Richard Sargent, two family practice physicians at the Family Health Clinic in Helena, Montana, unexpectedly gained national attention with some surprising research findings. They appear to be the first to demonstrate a direct link between a public smoking ban and an immediate decline in heart attacks. The doctors had never done medical research before, instead devoting their time to helping patients and keeping active in efforts to improve the public health of residents of their Montana town of 65,000 people. In recent years, they had worked for a ban on smoking in public places such as workplaces, restaurants, bowling alleys, bars, casinos, and truck stops—one of the strictest bans in the state and even the country.

Sometime after the ban began in June 2002, the two colleagues were having a conversation when Dr. Sargent mentioned that he had noticed a surprising drop in heart attacks. Could it be due to the smoking ordinance? Dr. Shepard was skeptical, but to see if the impression had any validity, he began to examine the medical records for the town's single hospital, St. Peter's Community Hospital. After weeding out cases involving those from outside the town, he found that during the four years preceding the ban, about 6.8 admissions for heart attacks occurred each month. During the time of the ban, there were 3 admissions each month—a drop of 56 percent. The drop occurred primarily among smokers but secondarily among nonsmokers. In December 2002, when the ban ended because a court ruling overturned its legality, heart attacks began to rise again. Shepard and Sargent consulted Stanton Glantz, a statistician and tobacco control expert at the University of California, San Francisco, who computed that the results could have occurred by chance only two out of one thousand times.

The study, presented at the annual meeting of the American College of Cardiology in Chicago in April 2003, demonstrates the immediate effect of reducing exposure of people to secondhand smoke. Given the size of the town examined, the study needs to be replicated in larger cities and states that have passed smoking bans. As Sargent acknowledges, "This is a tiny, little community in the middle of nowhere." Still, the results are intriguing. Although the harm of smoking is well known, few would have expected such large benefits so quickly. Averting 3 to 4 heart attacks a month, about 36 per year, would save millions of dollars for treatment of victims and untold suffering from the premature death of loved ones. As Shepard notes, "Neither of us ever dreamed we'd come to Helena, Montana, and make a significant contribution to the medical literature. We wouldn't have believed it."[34]

---

## Ending an Addiction

Despite the long-term gains to health, well-being, and finances from quitting smoking, immediate costs come from withdrawal symptoms caused by the body's continued need for the additive drug, nicotine. Viewed more positively, quitting smoking can eventually overcome an addiction that controls the life of a smoker.

In 1988, the surgeon general released a report bluntly stating that the "processes that determine tobacco addiction are similar to those that determine addiction to other drugs, including illegal drugs."[35] In general terms, addiction involves behavior that is controlled by a substance that causes changes in mood from its effects on the brain (unlike, say, for food that improves mood by meeting requirements for nourishment). Nicotine is such an addictive substance, causing changes in mood and compelling smokers to act in ways that damage themselves and society. Like addiction to hard drugs, addiction to nicotine produces uncomfortable withdrawal symptoms unless the smoker lights up again. Such addiction occurs not only from cigarettes but also from smokeless tobacco (and less so, from cigars and pipes) and the distribution of nicotine to the body through the mouth.

That many smokers quit successfully does not, according to the surgeon general, negate the claim of nicotine addiction. Spontaneous remission or unaided quitting occurs among 30 percent of hard drug users as well as smokers but leaves many others who face difficulties trying to end their dependence on the addictive substances. For both drugs and cigarettes, some people are more prone to becoming addicted than others and have a more difficult time quitting. Such variation occurs in most human behavior and simply means that susceptibility to cigarette addiction, if not universal, is at least common. Of course, cigarettes are legal, and most hard drugs are not. Hard drugs more than cigarettes negatively affect the ability of addicts to participate in daily life, increase the criminal actions associated with the habit, and produce more disgust in conventional society. Still, the control of one's actions by an artificial substance and the difficulty in ending the dependence on the substance make nicotine similar to hard drugs.

All this means that although most smokers and other tobacco users want to quit, they find the process difficult. Giving up tobacco causes strong cravings for the product that when not satisfied, produce irritability, restlessness, depression, anxiety, sleep disorder, and physical discomfort. People with these symptoms often have trouble concentrating on daily tasks. The withdrawal symptoms largely disappear after three to four weeks, but the cravings remain for much longer periods, sometimes indefinitely; former smokers often report that they miss the habit years after they have stopped. This continued attraction results not only from the physical dependence but also from the memory of the pleasurable feelings (stimulation of the mind and relaxation of the muscles) and behaviors (eating, drinking alcohol, socializing) associated with smoking and other tobacco use.

Consistent with the addiction framework and the difficulty in stopping smoking, smokers who are trying to quit have a high failure rate. In fact, 75 to 80 percent of quitters relapse within six months, and only 3 to 5 percent of smokers succeed in quitting for a year or more.[36] Yet, even the low rate of success, when accumulated over time, can do much to reduce smoking. Individuals who have failed to stop in the past may succeed in stopping with additional attempts. Thus, about 44 million Americans today are former smokers—roughly similar to the number of current smokers.

Preventing youth from ever starting to smoke obviously avoids the problems of overcoming nicotine addiction and does more for health than quitting. However, young people often start to smoke before they fully realize the extent of addictiveness of nicotine and the damages to the body brought on by smoking. Efforts to both prevent starting to smoke and end current smoking remain important.

## TRENDS IN TOBACCO USE

Use of cigarettes—the major form of tobacco consumption and the major cause of smoking-related illness—rose steadily from the late nineteenth century until the 1950s (see figure 6.1). In the 1950s, consumption leveled off and even declined briefly after publicity from several popular reports about the harm of cigarettes for lung cancer. However, consumption again rose in the late 1950s and peaked in 1963. The famous report of the surgeon general on health and smoking published in 1964 bluntly told people interested in their health and a long life to give up smoking. Given the desire of nearly all people to avoid dying early, it would seem that the mounting evidence against smoking would lead to the disappearance of the habit. The percentage of the U.S. population that smoked did indeed decline, as did the overall consumption of cigarettes, but not as fast as public health advocates would have liked. Reviewing the trends, the 1989 surgeon general's report could point to substantial progress.[37] The yearly number of cigarettes consumed per adult fell from 3,910 in 1963 to 2,724 in 1990. From 1965 to 1990, the percentage of male smokers fell from 51.9 percent to 28.4, and the percentage of female smokers fell from 33.9 percent to 22.8 percent (see figure 6.2). The decline among males exceeded that among females in large part because males started at higher levels. Despite a greater decline in smoking among light and moderate smokers, who were less addicted to nicotine than heavy smokers, the trends encouraged public health officials.

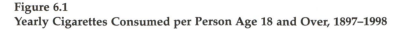

**Figure 6.1**
**Yearly Cigarettes Consumed per Person Age 18 and Over, 1897–1998**

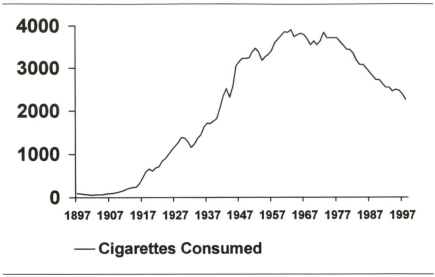

— **Cigarettes Consumed**

*Source:* U.S. Bureau of the Census, *Historical Statistics of the United States, Colonial Times to 1970* (Washington, D.C.: Department of Commerce, 1973); and U.S. Bureau of the Census, *Statistical Abstract* (Washington, D.C.: U.S. Department of Commerce, various years).

Smoking among youth declined much as it did for older groups from the mid-1960s to 1990. Because youth smoking leads to addiction and foretells future trends at older ages, progress against smoking at these ages had special importance. For young adults age 18 to 24, male smoking prevalence fell from 54 percent in 1965 to 25 percent in 1990, and female smoking prevalence fell from 37 to 22 percent over the same period. Yearly surveys of high school seniors, which began in 1976, reveal a similar decline in daily smoking until 1990 (see figure 6.3). For boys, such smoking fell from 38 percent to 29 percent, and for girls, it fell from 39 percent to 29 percent.

The optimism that greeted these advances did not last through the 1990s, however. Although some encouraging signs continued, the rate of decline in cigarette smoking slowed (see figure 6.2). Among adults from 1990 to 1998, the percentages of current male smokers fell by only 2 percent—from 28.4 percent to 26.4 percent.[38] For females, the decline was even smaller, falling from 22.8 percent to 22.0 percent. Among smokers in the 1990s, light and moderate consumption of cigarettes increased relative to heavy smoking, but with no smoking better than any smoking, the

**Figure 6.2**
**Trends in Percentage Current Smokers and Percentage Ever Smokers for Men and Women, 1965–1998**

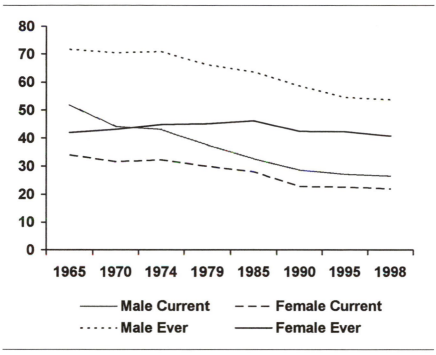

*Source:* U.S. Department of Health and Human Services, *Women and Smoking: A Report of the Surgeon General* (Rockville, Md.: U.S. Department of Health and Human Services, Public Health Service, Office of the Surgeon General, 2001), pp. 34–37.

percentages appear discouragingly slow to change. Overall, after some 35 years of antismoking efforts, about one-quarter of the U.S. adult population continues with the habit. Given the population of the United States, these percentages translate into roughly 40–50 million current smokers and about an equal number of former smokers.

The trends among young people during the 1990s offered no more encouragement. Rather than falling, smoking in fact showed some increases. From 1990 to 1998, current smoking among young men ages 18–24 rose from 25.1 to 31.5 percent, and current smoking among young women rose from 22.4 to 25.1 percent. Among high school seniors, the trends show a disconcerting rise from a low point in 1992 of 26 percent for girls and 29 percent for boys to 34 percent for girls and 36 percent for boys in 1998 (see figure 6.3). Since then, however, smoking among high school seniors

**Figure 6.3**
**Trends in Percentage Current Smokers for Male and Female High School Seniors, 1976–1998**

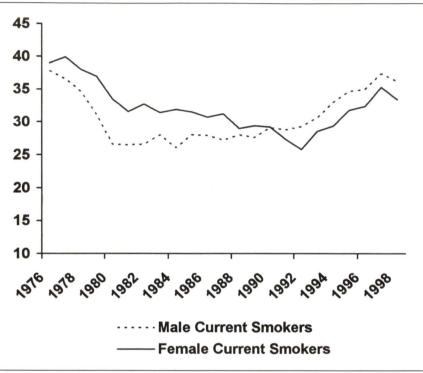

······ **Male Current Smokers**
——— **Female Current Smokers**

*Source:* U.S. Department of Health and Human Services, *Women and Smoking: A Report of the Surgeon General* (Rockville, Md.: U.S. Department of Health and Human Services, Public Health Service, Office of the Surgeon General, 2001), p. 60.

has fallen each year, and most hope that the trend will continue downward. In any case, the rise and then fall leave current levels of smoking about the same today as a decade ago.[39]

Cigars have for most of the last half century declined in popularity but have enjoyed resurgent popularity in the 1990s. In 1970, 16.2 percent of men smoked cigars. The figure fell to 3.5 percent by 1991 but rose to 8.4 percent in 1998 (female cigar smoking remained negligible). The resurgence of cigar smoking relates to the desire to enjoy their flavor and aroma, much as one enjoys gourmet food and quality liquor. The largest increase has thus come in the consumption of premium cigars, particularly among white males ages 25 to 34. Although for most, cigar smoking involves an occasional pleasure rather than a daylong habit, the health risks faced by occasional cigar smokers are greater than for those who abstain altogether from tobacco products.[40]

Smokeless tobacco use also failed to decline in the 1990s, staying at 5 to 6 percent among men (female use is again negligible). Pipe smoking has declined among men after a brief period of popularity in the 1960s. Use of bidis, a tobacco product common in India but new to the United States, has increased among youth. Bidis are small, brown cigarettes that are hand rolled in a leaf and tied at one end by a string. About 4 percent of girls and 12 percent of boys have tried the product, but few use it on a regular basis.

Antismoking forces, public health experts, and government agencies have worked hard to lessen tobacco use in the population and have discovered some effective ways to move toward this goal. Initial efforts involved disseminating information on the dangers of smoking, but education alone seldom proves sufficient to overcome the attractions to the habit. Government regulatory efforts have had more success. These include limiting advertising and promotion of cigarettes targeted at children and youth, banning smoking in public buildings, enforcing laws to prevent minors from purchasing cigarettes, and sponsoring litigation against tobacco companies. Perhaps most effectively, government-imposed taxes increase the costs of cigarettes and reduce the consumption of the product. Comprehensive school, community, state, and media-based antismoking programs can also postpone or prevent smoking onset in 20 to 40 percent of adolescents but are not common.[41]

## CIGARETTES IN THE MOVIES

In 1999, the American Lung Association gave its Thumbs Down Award to the popular comedy movie *There's Something about Mary* for having the two lead characters smoke cigarettes and placing Kool brand cigarettes in numerous scenes. The two stars, Ben Stiller and Cameron Diaz, received Dishonorable Mentions for both lighting up during a romantic scene. The blockbuster movie *Armageddon* received the association's Thumbs Up Award because the characters, Bruce Willis and Liv Tyler in particular, do not use tobacco, even when facing likely doom for the earth and themselves.[42]

With tobacco companies forced by litigation to eliminate advertising targeted at youth and to stop associating smoking with glamour, sexuality, and sophistication, the promotion of tobacco in films has become an important substitute for advertising. For example, Meg Ryan, Rene Zellweger, Winona Ryder, Gwyneth Paltrow, and Catherine Zeta-Jones have all used cigarettes in recent film roles. As models for teens, these actors can have much influence on the willingness of young girls to start smoking.

A review of the top 25 box-office films for each year from 1988 to 1997 found that more than 85 percent of the films contained tobacco use.[43] Nearly as many instances of tobacco use occurred in movies for adolescents (PG and PG-13) as in movies for adults (R). Worse, "there were more than twice as many scenes that glorified tobacco use as put it down," and movies rarely tried "to depict smoking and other tobacco use in its true light with actors coughing and hacking and having stained teeth."[44] Antismoking advocates have called for Hollywood to take steps to avoid glamorizing smoking.

## SMOKING AND PROGRESS AGAINST HEART DISEASE

Lower rates of smoking appear to have contributed importantly to the decline in heart disease mortality during the 1960s and 1970s.[45] In one study for the years 1968 to 1981, a period when heart disease mortality decreased, substantial declines in smoking occurred, from 51 percent in 1965 to 36 percent in 1980 for men and 33 percent to 29 percent for women.[46] For a slightly shorter period, another study concludes that "reductions in smoking levels may have accounted for about 24 percent of the decline in coronary mortality between 1968 and 1976."[47]

However, the decline in mortality from heart disease involves more than smoking. Since death rates have fallen among both smokers and nonsmokers, other factors besides tobacco use must contribute to the progress against heart disease.[48] Moreover, the slower decline in smoking in the last decade does not match the continuing steady decline in heart disease. Estimates accordingly suggest that stopping smoking accounted for only 6 percent of the decline in deaths from 1980 to 1990.[49] A more recent study of nurses from 1980 to 1994 attributes somewhat more importance to smoking.[50] It finds that the incidence of coronary disease among the sample declined by 31 percent during this time period for this sample, with smoking explaining about 13 percent of the decline. Despite these results, preventing heart disease through stopping smoking remains crucial—the problem has been that the success of antismoking efforts has stalled recently.

Even if changes in smoking have not done much in recent years to reduce heart disease, the potential for future improvement remains. Further declines in smoking will come with more difficulty than in the past, but they appear possible. Estimates suggest that comprehensive state programs can reduce adult smoking prevalence by about 1 percent per year. At that pace, the Healthy People 2010 goal of 15 percent smoking prevalence can be reached or even bettered.[51] Tobacco control efforts—litigation, higher taxes, policies to ban smoking, controls on advertising to youth, and advances in smoking cessation—have potential for success. And further declines in tobacco use can contribute to future declines in mortality. Such antitobacco efforts can do much to reduce heart disease in the early part of the twenty-first century.

# CHAPTER 7

# Diet and Exercise

On June 20, 2002, President George W. Bush announced a new program to promote a healthier lifestyle for Americans. Named HealthierUSA, the initiative focuses on four areas in which the average American, regardless of age or sex, could improve health through good decision making and lifestyle choices. The initiative's four-pronged approach encourages Americans to be physically active every day, eat a nutritious diet, get preventative screenings, and make healthy choices. Citing findings and statistics from the Department of Health and Human Services, President Bush made clear the positive effect basic changes in lifestyle could have on the overall health of the American people and on the costs associated with treating chronic disease. For example, the Bush administration estimated that if 10 percent of adults began walking regularly, Americans could save $5.6 billion in costs linked to heart disease. Another statistic cited by the government showed that Americans pay for their sedentary lifestyles with an estimated $117 billion annually in problems associated with obesity and overweight alone.[1]

The president's approach to promoting fitness and health matches the basic opinions held by most medical professionals today. If people know they are at risk because of behavioral patterns (smoking, not exercising, eating too much junk food, etc.), they can take steps to address the potential problems before they turn into frightening, debilitating, or life-threatening events. This is the goal of the HealthierUSA initiative and explains why it promotes simple and inexpensive behavioral changes designed to favor quality-of-life increases and reduced economic costs for those at risk or living with chronic diseases. Modest exercise, as little as a half hour spent walking, can prevent many chronic diseases. For example, a brisk 30-minute walk can use 150–200 calories (depending on one's weight). Done daily, it lowers weight, reduces blood pressure, and improves heart rate. More strenuous exercise may bring even greater benefits.

Likewise, most Americans can achieve good overall nutrition through simple adjustments to diet—such as increasing fruit and vegetable consumption and avoiding both fried foods and excessive portions—and help lower the risk not only of heart disease but also of stroke, cancer, and osteoporosis. Preventative screening takes only a visit to the doctor, and avoiding tobacco, drug, and alcohol abuse is a lifestyle choice each person has the ability to make.

Heart disease likewise can be prevented or managed, to a large extent, by the way one chooses to live. If the White House initiative results in more Americans eating healthier diets and increasing their exercise to combat the growing problem of overweight and obesity, heart disease likely will continue to decline and Americans will live longer, healthier lives. This goal also requires people to educate themselves about the risks of heart disease and how to decrease these risks.

Actor and director Stephen Furst, "Flounder" from the classic film *Animal House,* had many risk factors for heart disease, including obesity and diabetes, and he maintained a diet high in saturated fat, consuming a lot of junk food and fast food that lacked nutritional balance. His lifestyle was too sedentary, and he could not exercise enough to use up all the calories he consumed each day. Furthermore, he was genetically predisposed to diabetes: his father died of a diabetes-related heart attack at age 47, the same year Furst, at 17, was diagnosed with type 2 diabetes. Type 2 diabetes is the result of insulin resistance (when the body does not use insulin to break down blood sugars properly) and general insulin deficiency. It is the most common type of diabetes, affecting approximately 95 percent of all 17 million diabetes sufferers in the United States.[2] Also known as adult-onset diabetes (though studies show the average age at which it appears has dropped significantly over recent years), it is associated, much like heart disease, with obesity, a sedentary lifestyle, and genetics. Heart disease is in fact one of the worst complications of diabetes. Furst ignored the diagnosis for 25 years, until the late 1990s, and was lucky to survive without having to face any of the serious complications that could arise. During this time, he remained seriously overweight, at his heaviest, about 320 pounds. Then, he was hospitalized because of a diabetes-related incident. A blister on his foot became infected and, because of poor blood circulation from his diabetes, he risked losing the foot. Fortunately, he recovered, but the incident scared him and led him to change his lifestyle.

Furst focused his lifestyle-change effort on specific areas that he knew could improve his health: he concentrated on cooking and eating nutritional foods and eating smaller portions. He also began exercising regularly. Now, he maintains a healthy weight of about 175 pounds, he no longer requires insulin for his diabetes, and his risk for heart disease has dropped dramatically. He has become a spokesperson for the American Heart Association, helping to educate people about diabetes and heart disease through humor and a willingness to talk about his own experiences.[3]

## BACKGROUND

In 1948, the National Heart Institute (today known as the National Heart, Lung, and Blood Institute) and the American Heart Association were established. That year, the federal government funneled approximately $500,000 into heart research.[4] Because no intensive research had been conducted previously, evidence pointing to a causal relationship between blood cholesterol levels and coronary heart disease had not been gathered, nor was hypercholesterolemia (very high blood cholesterol) believed to be abnormal. However, geographic differences in rates of cardiovascular heart disease provided possible clues.[5] In subsequent years, major studies defined the way the medical community has approached and understood heart disease ever since. The late 1940s and early 1950s marked the beginning of a period when the U.S. government as well as individual researchers and the international medical community became more seriously committed to research projects focused on heart disease. Given the epidemic rise of heart disease, understanding its causes and developing preventative care and treatment plans became important objectives. From the beginning, much of this research pointed to cultural and behavioral risk factors such as diet, fitness, and smoking. This was significant because it meant to a large extent that prevention and treatment of heart disease could be addressed through behavioral changes and education, instead of costly medical procedures or medication.

Today, many people take for granted the knowledge that certain behaviors increase their risk of developing disease. Some risk factors, such as smoking, are accepted by almost everyone as likely to cause early death and other health problems. A large part of this is the result of successful public education and advocacy campaigns resulting in greater awareness. For heart disease, the risks related to smoking, high blood pressure, and cholesterol are fairly well known by most, although many of the finer points have not been adequately or clearly enough expressed. Other risk factors for heart disease, such as a sedentary lifestyle and obesity, are only now gaining popular notice. These risk factors have been apparent for a long time now, since the late 1960s and early 1970s, but recent studies have increased our understanding of how they relate to heart disease and the actual costs and degree of risk associated with them. The studies that first found these risks were conducted after the end of World War II, and much progress against heart disease and other chronic diseases stems from the knowledge gained from the early studies.

The cross-country comparisons of Ancel Keys's epidemiological investigation (population study) into cardiovascular disease and the Framingham study funded and operated by the National Heart Institute were the first to establish the major risk factors for cardiovascular heart disease. Both studies found that high blood cholesterol, high blood pressure, smoking, and dietary factors such as cholesterol, fat, and sodium were major risk factors associated with heart disease.[6] Keys's "Seven Countries Study" (initiated in 1958 and continuing through today) and his study of Minnesota businessmen (which he started several months before the Framingham study began) showed that bloodstream cholesterol was the chief determinant of heart disease. He also found other risk factors that existed, such as hypertension and smoking. His studies revealed that saturated fat in the diet was a chief determinant of cholesterol in the blood, and he illustrated that a whole population could be at high risk of early death based on their diet and exercise practices.[7]

The Framingham study was a 20-year project that followed five thousand men and women aged 32 to 60 living in Framingham, Massachusetts, who did not have signs of heart disease when the study began. The subjects were checked every two years for signs or symptoms of heart disease. The Framingham study was the first to show that the higher the blood cholesterol level the greater the likelihood that a person will develop coronary heart disease. Over the years, the research suggested that several other risk factors were also associated with heart disease, including socioeconomic status, obesity, exercise, smoking, elevated blood pressure, male gender, and high blood-sugar levels, to name a few. During the two decades the study spanned, it played a leading role in heart research, providing important insight into strokes and heart attacks as well as heart disease. Along with Keys's studies, the Framingham study acted as the foundation on which future studies built, and much of the progress against heart disease during the twentieth century stems from these early studies. Thanks to discoveries of Keys and the Framingham study, heart disease became a "hot" topic and an important public health concern. Current foci of research, including diet and exercise, descend from these first studies.

The Framingham and Keys studies were not the only ones to tackle heart disease. In the 1950s, John Gofman and colleagues began to investigate lipoprotein patterns, ultimately finding a correlation between concentrations of certain classes of lipoproteins and the incidence of coronary heart disease.[8] This study first brought attention to the correlation between high levels of LDL and risk of coronary heart disease and the inverse correlation between levels of HDL and risk of coronary heart disease. LDL cholesterol is commonly known as "bad cholesterol." It contributes to buildup of plaque in the arteries. Over time, the plaque deposits create a blockage, preventing blood from flowing through the arteries. Ruptured plaque may also block the flow of blood to the heart. HDL cholesterol is also known as "good cholesterol." It moves through the blood and picks up cholesterol to transport it to the liver for destruction.

In the 1970s, heart studies confirmed that high blood levels of HDL correspond to a reduced risk of developing coronary heart disease.[9] A person's ratio of LDL to HDL, measured through a common blood test, is now looked at as a primary indicator of risk for coronary heart disease. In 1981, research results published from an Oslo heart study showed people could improve their heart's health simply by eating a better diet and quitting smoking.[10] The existence of a direct link between high blood cholesterol levels and heart disease was confirmed further in 1984 by the Lipid Research Clinics Coronary Primary Prevention Trial. This trial showed that lowering LDL, bad cholesterol, significantly lowers the risk of developing heart disease.[11]

In 1993, the then deputy assistant secretary for health (J. Michael McGinnis) and the former director of the Centers for Disease Control and Prevention (William Foege) coauthored a journal article, "Actual Causes of Death in the U.S." They concluded that a combination of dietary factors and sedentary activity patterns then accounted for at least 300,000 deaths each year, the second-leading cause of preventable death in the United States behind tobacco use.[12] This study helped establish public health priorities and played an important role in directing research toward where it is today.

So where are we in terms of understanding heart disease today? We know diet and exercise play a highly significant role in putting people at risk for developing coronary heart disease. Perhaps more important, we know they are extremely important behavioral factors in maintaining a healthy heart and in reversing some of the symptoms of heart disease. Still, there is much to learn. The good news regarding funding for the fiscal year 2003 was that the Senate Appropriations Committee earmarked approximately $2.8 billion for the research at the National Heart, Lung, and Blood Institute.[13] Much of this money will go into further research on risk factors for heart disease, as they relate both to behavioral and medical strategies for prevention and treatment. This focus on risk factors stems from the concrete results seen by physicians indicating a drop in heart disease for patients who follow therapeutic programs designed to decrease risk factors.

The rest of this chapter deals primarily with the risk factors associated with diet and physical activity. The major aspects of diet are discussed, providing definitions for each and then a brief treatment of dangers and strategies for facing the dangers. After diet, exercise is examined. Finally, the issues of overweight and obesity, which are integrally related to life-style patterns of diet and exercise and are a major area of interest today, are covered.

## ANCEL KEYS, PIONEERING HEART SCIENTIST

Ancel Keys was born on January 26, 1904, in Colorado Springs, Colorado. Just before the great earthquake and fire of 1906, he and his family moved to San Francisco, where he grew up. An uncle, Lon Chaney, was a silent film star in Hollywood.

A successful student, Keys received his bachelor's degree from Berkeley in 1925 and by 1930 had earned a doctorate in oceanography and biology. In 1938, he completed a second doctorate, in physiology, at Cambridge University in England. Keys became a professor at the University of Minnesota in 1936, where he established the Laboratory of Physiological Hygiene, which he directed from 1939 until his retirement in 1975. Over several decades, he played an important role in establishing modern cardiovascular disease epidemiology and bringing to light fundamental issues about the way diet and exercise affect human physiology.

In 1941, the U.S. Army asked Keys to develop a compact, lightweight, and highly nutritious meal for combat troops. The meal became known as K-rations and consisted of biscuits, canned meat, chocolate, and powdered coffee or lemonade. Cigarettes, matches, and toilet paper were added later by the army.

During World War II, Keys studied starvation and subsistence diets. Some of the research was conducted on conscientious objectors to the war who volunteered for the study. They endured regulated, near-starvation diets, and their physiological responses to lack of nutrition were recorded in detail. The study was intended to provide insight into the health of war-ravaged populations in postwar Europe. Keys compiled his findings in the two-volume *Biology of Human Starvation* (1950), which showed, among other insights, that changes in diet had a profound affect on physiological health. He also noticed, around this time, that presumably well fed American business executives had high rates of heart attacks while postwar Europeans, who had been under severe diet restrictions from war rationing, showed sharply decreased rates of cardiovascular disease. This led Keys to believe there was a correlation between cholesterol levels and heart problems, so he began the first prospective study of cardiovascular disease in 1947, with a sample of Minnesota businessmen. This led him to undertake further studies, culminating in the Seven Countries Study, which, since 1958, has followed a sample of men from distinct populations who live in seven countries in North America, Europe, and Asia. By looking at whole populations, he established that diet and activity are the major factors in determining the risk of heart disease.

When the Seven Countries Study results were first published in 1970, Keys found strong associations between the coronary heart disease rate of a population and average blood cholesterol and per capita intake of saturated fat. In other words, he had shown that diets high in saturated fat result in high cholesterol levels while diets low in saturated fats lead to low cholesterol. These findings caused something of a cholesterol controversy to erupt, with scientists split over whether statistically "strong associations" provided scientific certainty. Interventionists, like Keys, argued that the epidemiological studies provided enough certainty to begin reevaluation of treatment and diagnosis immediately. Those on the other side of the debate wanted further studies before taking action—preferably clinical or laboratory studies. Keys also found tobacco was a major risk fact of heart disease along with high blood pressure.

In the years that have followed since those early studies were completed, Keys and his wife Margaret have promoted the benefits of reasonably low fat diets. Their popular cookbooks, including *Eat Well, Stay Well the Mediterranean Way* and *The Benevolent Bean*, describe the value of the of the Mediterranean diet and lifestyle, combining science with practical suggestions for cooking and eating a tasty, low-fat diet. Changes in the U.S. diet and the downward trend in heart disease in America over the last 50 years are due in good part to this pioneering scientist.[14]

## DIET

People with a diet low in total fat, saturated fat, cholesterol, and sodium are more likely to maintain a healthy heart than those who regularly eat food high in any or all of these categories. For a healthy heart as well as a healthy body, the U.S. Food and Drug Administration recommends that Americans eat less fat and sodium; reduce their caloric intake if they are overweight; eat more fiber and eat a variety of foods; eat plenty of bread, rice, cereal, and fruits and vegetables; and, if they drink alcohol, do so in moderation.[15] The Food and Drug Administration also urges Americans to pay attention to their cholesterol and consult with a doctor about cholesterol levels. Generally, levels less than 200 mg/dL are desirable; levels between 200 mg/dL and 239 mg/dL are borderline high; and 240 mg/dL and above are high.[16] High cholesterol levels usually indicate high risk for heart disease.

### Cholesterol

Cholesterol is found in animal products, including cheese, meat, dairy, butter, and eggs. Vegetables and their oils, grains, and nuts and seeds do not contain cholesterol because it does not occur in plants. The human liver produces most of the cholesterol we need to survive; however, our bodies also take cholesterol from the food we eat. The daily recommended limit of dietary cholesterol is 300 mg. For people who are cholesterol-sensitive, consuming more than this amount regularly can raise cholesterol levels. About one in three Americans are sensitive to cholesterol in their diets.[17] People with high cholesterol are at a higher risk of developing heart disease than those who maintain lower levels. This is because excess cholesterol clogs arteries and causes atherosclerosis.

Many doctors believe the ratio of bad to good cholesterol (LDL/HDL) is a more important risk factor than actual cholesterol levels. LDLs are particles that transport cholesterol into the cells. Optimal LDL cholesterol levels are less than 100 mg/dL, while more than 160 is considered high or very high. For HDL cholesterol, higher levels indicate less risk. HDL levels below 40 mg/dL are low, and levels above 60 mg/dL help lower the risk of heart disease.[18] It is believed that oxidized LDL cholesterol is particularly threatening because, more than other types, it seems prone to attaching itself to inflamed tissue. Oxidized LDL is found in many processed foods, as well as in much of the food available in fast-food restaurants. Elements known as free radicals attack LDL, thus oxidizing it. For this reason, many people believed antioxidants such as vitamin E may benefit the body by reducing free radicals and preventing the oxidization of LDL. Recent studies suggest that while vitamins may promote overall health, antioxidants do not seem to help those with heart disease lower their risk and may in fact interfere with some of the most often prescribed cholesterol-lowering drugs.[19]

Many people who have not shown risk from cholesterol have lethal or debilitating heart events, and many others who have high cholesterol do not have problems with their heart. More important than the amount of cholesterol one consumes may be the types of foods containing the cholesterol.

## Triglycerides and Fats

Fats are found in much of the food we eat. There are four main types we consume: saturated fat, polyunsaturated fat, monounsaturated fat, and trans-fatty acids (trans-fats). Saturated fats are made up of carbon and hydrogen, with the carbon holding as many hydrogens as it is able. Saturated fat is usually solid at room temperature, does not bond easily with oxygen, and most often comes from animal products. Unsaturated fats are fats that have open bonds where hydrogen could attach itself. Polyunsaturated fats, which come from many plant oils including safflower, sesame, soy, corn, and sunflower as well as from nuts and seeds, are liquid at room temperature and in the refrigerator. Monounsaturated fats, coming from sources like olive oil, canola and peanut oil, and avocados, are liquid at room temperature and begin to solidify in the refrigerator. Trans-fats are a kind of unsaturated fat that hydrogen has been added to for cooking (hydrogenated or partially hydrogenated vegetable oil). It shows up in many deep-fried, commercially baked, and processed foods. Saturated fats and trans-fats have been shown to increase cholesterol levels. Poly-unsaturated fats assist the body in disposing of newly formed cholesterol, helping to clear the artery walls of cholesterol and making the blood less congested. Monounsaturated fats may also help, to a limited degree, in reducing cholesterol. People who eat a diet high in saturated fats are at a much higher risk of developing heart disease than those who eat mostly unsaturated fats. Saturated fats, especially hard fats like those commonly found in lard, raise LDL cholesterol. On the other hand, unsaturated vege-table fats tend to lower LDL and raise HDL cholesterol. Both saturated and unsaturated fats should be consumed in moderation.

Triglycerides are the chemical form taken by most fats. When a person eats, whatever calories are not quickly used the body convert into tri-glycerides for storage in fat cells. Hormones then regulate the release of triglycerides for use as energy during the periods between meals. Elevated triglyceride levels are linked to heart and blood vessel disease in some people and can be the result of other conditions, such as untreated dia-betes. Triglyceride levels can be tested for in the same way that cholesterol is, through a simple blood test.

### Omega-3 Fatty Acids and Phytochemicals

Omega-3 fatty acids are found in fish and fish oils as well as certain types of vegetables. They are known to help keep the heart healthy in people without heart disease as well as improve the health of those with heart disease. Fatty fishes such as salmon, mackerel, and albacore tuna contain two important types of omega-3 fatty acids. Soy, canola, walnut, and flax-seed oils also contain an omega-3 fatty acid that is less potent than those found in fish oils but still helpful to the heart. Omega-3 fatty acids have been shown in studies to decrease inflammation, balance the immune system, slow down blood clotting, lower blood lipids and pos-sibly cholesterol, and have a stabilizing effect on the heart rhythm.[20] And although the mechanisms responsible for omega-3 fatty acids' reduction of coronary heart disease risk are not completely understood, research has shown that omega-3 fatty acids lower risk of sudden death and arrhyth-mia; decrease the risk of thrombosis (blood clot); reduce triglyceride lev-els; impair growth of atherosclerotic plaque, the buildup that can cause heart attacks; improve overall arterial health; and lower blood pressure.[21]

Fruits and vegetables also contain micronutrients call phytochemicals. They are broken into several categories including plant sterols (including stanols), flavonoids, and plant-sulfur compounds. Many of these phyto-chemicals show promise for reducing the risk of atherosclerosis. Some have been studied in the past, and others are only recently being studied, but all need more research to understand better exactly how they may help the heart.

## Types of Recommended Diets

The results of recent research have led many institutions concerned with the health of Americans to suggest dietary guidelines for a healthy heart, good overall nutrition, and preventing obesity. There is substantial evidence "that diets using nonhydrogenated unsaturated fats as the predominant form of dietary fat, whole grains as the main form of carbohydrates, an abundance of fruit and vegetables, and adequate omega-3 fatty acids can offer significant protection against coronary heart disease. Such diets, together with regular physical activity, avoidance of smoking, and maintenance of a health body weight, may prevent the majority of cardiovascular disease in Western populations."[22] Likewise, a recent study in Canada suggests that a specialized vegetarian diet containing a high percentage of soy and soluble fiber may reduce cholesterol by two to three times the amount that most people can expect through other dietary changes.[23] This particular diet, although promising, requires confirmation and replication in the world outside the laboratory.

The Mediterranean diet that Ancel Keys favored, the hunter-gatherer diet (also called prehistoric), and the diet that is loosely tied to the U.S. Department of Agriculture's (USDA) food pyramid guidelines, recommended by the American Heart Association, the National Heart, Lung, and Blood Institute, and other government agencies, have received considerable attention. These diets, as well as the soy diet already mentioned, have common elements of low saturated fat and relatively high complex carbohydrates. These diets, with variations, work on the premise that eating foods low in cholesterol (no more than 30 percent of your calories should be from fat, and 10 percent or less from saturated fat and trans-fatty acids) will keep LDL levels within a safe range.

Many Americans follow some variation of the American Heart Association's two-tiered recommended diet meant to help virtually all Americans age two and older. Step one is supposed to improve the overall health and reduce the risk of heart disease in most Americans. Step two is more intensive and rigid for those who have tried step one without adequate results.[24]

Step one of the American Heart Association diet emphasizes the importance of maintaining appropriate body weight, which can be determined from height-weight tables or the body-mass index, to achieve health because overweight and obesity are major risks for cardiovascular disease. To help avoid obesity as well as elevated blood cholesterol, 30 percent or less of daily calories from fat is recommended. Less than 10 percent of total calories should come from saturated fat, which increases blood cholesterol levels in susceptible individuals, and unsaturated fats are preferable because they lower blood cholesterol levels without lowering HDL (good) cholesterol. Eating fatty fish, as long as it has not been deep fried or cooked with saturated fats, is also recommended because of the omega-3 fatty acids it contains that help lower LDL (bad) cholesterol.

The guidelines for the step-one diet also deal with other factors. For those who drink alcohol, moderation is key, with a recommended limit of no more than the equivalent of two glasses of wine or two 12-ounce beers each day. Drinkers should know that alcohol consumed in small amounts appears to help lower cholesterol and reduce atherosclerosis to a limited degree. One to two drinks per day may help lower the risk of heart disease by as much as 30 to 40 percent.[25] Alcohol appears to help raise levels of HDL cholesterol and thin the blood, reducing the chance of blood clots that can block the flow of blood to the heart. The step-one diet does not promote the idea that nondrinkers should begin drinking, nor does it endorse the use of alcohol by pregnant women or others whose health may be affected negatively by even small amounts of alcohol, like alcoholics.

Sodium consumption is a serious concern. The amount one consumes per day should not exceed 2,400 mg, or less than one teaspoon of table salt. Diets high in sodium can result in hypertension, which is a known risk factor for heart disease. Five servings of vegetables and fruits daily is the target for keeping the heart and blood vessels healthy through the step-one diet, and eating a variety of vegetables and fruits is a good idea. Dark-green leafy vegetables, such as spinach, and orange or yellow vegetables, such as sweet potatoes and squash, are particularly nutrient rich. Nonetheless, as of the year 2000, less than 25 percent of American adults consumed the recommended amount of fruits and vegetables.[26] Finally, complex carbohydrates constituting at least 55 percent of total daily calories can be gained by eating at least six servings of grains, cereals, and lentils each day.

The step-two program, based on the same principles as the step-one diet, has been modified to more stringent standards. Instead of total dietary fat being 30 percent or less of daily calories, as in the step-one program, the step-two diet limits dietary fat to less than 30 percent of total calories. More rigid than the step-one program, step-two targets less than 7 percent of total calories from saturated fat (compared with no more than 10 percent in step one) and cholesterol consumption at less than 200 mg per day, or one-third less than step one.

Dietary changes can reduce blood levels of cholesterol within a month, and the levels can continue to drop over several months if the diet is maintained. Approximately 75 percent of Americans with high levels of cholesterol in their blood can be expected to decrease their cholesterol levels 10 to 15 percent with a change in their diet. Decreasing total cholesterol levels by 10 percent may result in a reduced incidence of coronary heart disease by as much as 30 percent.[27] Adding a regimen of moderate exercise to a low-fat, low-cholesterol diet enhances the effects of the diet on lowering blood cholesterol.

The American Heart Association's most recent revised guidelines for heart-healthy dietary practices move away from trying to balance Americans' diets by stating what each meal should and should not include. Instead, the new approach is based on general principles. In brief, the American Heart Association plan focuses on reducing fat intake, especially animal fats because they tend to raise cholesterol and thus increase the risk of heart and blood vessel disease. Overall, people who consume less fat have lower cholesterol levels and better ratios of LDL to HDL cholesterol. Indeed, diets extremely low in all fats—less than 10 percent— have been found to reduce the size of atherosclerotic plaque.[28]

While lifestyle can help control cholesterol levels, the link between dietary fat intake and heart disease may also have a genetic component. According to one recent study, based on a group of individuals over age 55 participating in the Framingham Offspring Study, those who have a specific mutation in a certain gene have the greatest risk for heart disease. This particular gene helps explain why some people are less successful than others in adapting to a Western high-fat diet.[29]

---

## THE USDA FOOD PYRAMID AND HOW TO USE IT

You can use the USDA food pyramid along with label information on foods to evaluate your eating habits and, if you want, to act on recommendations for Americans to follow healthy eating habits.[30] The food pyramid provides a basic outline of what to eat each day and how much to eat. It is not a rigid dietary plan, and people should modify how they use it according to their own circumstances. A doctor or nutritionist can help you plan a diet that is right for you. The main thing the food pyramid helps people see is that they do not have to avoid foods high in sodium, high in cholesterol, and high in fat *completely*, but they should eat foods that are high in these in small to moderate amounts, along with a wide variety of other foods that are low in these elements or missing them altogether. On food labels or boxes, words such as "free," "low" or "reduced" can signal right away that the food may be a good option for moderating consumption of these nutrients. In the same way, where you see "good source" or "high," look closer to see if they are describing dietary elements like fiber, vitamins and minerals that you need. (See figure 7.1.)

The health claims put on packaging of foods or labels are regulated by the Food and Drug Administration, so you can usually trust them, but inspect the nutrient facts label to make sure you know all the facts. For example, many foods may say "fat free" or "cholesterol free" on the packaging. While these health claims are true, they do not always give you the whole story. For example, many candies say "fat free," but they are extremely high

**Figure 7.1**
**USDA Food Pyramid**

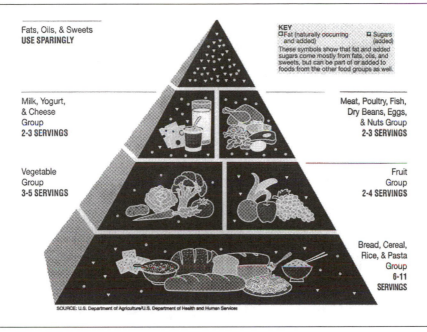

Fats, Oils, & Sweets
**USE SPARINGLY**

KEY
☐ Fat (naturally occurring     ▨ Sugars
and added)                        (added)
These symbols show that fat and added sugars come mostly from fats, oils, and sweets, but can be part of or added to foods from the other food groups as well.

Milk, Yogurt,
& Cheese
Group
**2-3 SERVINGS**

Meat, Poultry, Fish,
Dry Beans, Eggs,
& Nuts Group
**2-3 SERVINGS**

Vegetable
Group
**3-5 SERVINGS**

Fruit
Group
**2-4 SERVINGS**

Bread, Cereal,
Rice, & Pasta
Group
**6-11
SERVINGS**

SOURCE: U.S. Department of Agriculture/U.S. Department of Health and Human Services

*Source:* U.S. Department of Agriculture, "Food Pyramid," http://www.nalusda.gov/fnic/Fpyr/pyramid.gif (accessed May 2003).

in sugar, which will be stored as fat if you fail to use as much energy as you gain from eating it. And popcorn may be cholesterol free, sodium free, and low in fat, but most people cook popcorn in oil (fat) and cover it with butter (cholesterol) and salt (sodium).

Check out the part of the label that lists daily values of ingredients. These figures are based on a diet of 2,000 calories per day, which is roughly the amount moderately active women, teenage girls, and sedentary men require.

The food pyramid can help you follow the USDA dietary guidelines for planning a nutritious, well-balanced diet; eating a variety of foods; maintaining a healthy weight; regulating intake of cholesterol, fats, and added sugars; and controlling sodium consumption.[31] However, one point about diet is also worth remembering—ideas and science change. For example, the popular low-carbohydrate, high-fat and protein diet recommended for weight loss by Dr. Robert C. Atkins has for decades been heavily criticized for raising cholesterol. To the surprise of most of the medical establishment, recent research has found that the Atkins diet actually lowers blood lipids.[32] Questions about the diet remain, and most cardiologists are hesitant to recommend it. Still, the preliminary evidence is intriguing.

## EXERCISE

Regular exercise—including walking, swimming, gardening, and jogging—is an important factor for keeping a healthy heart. Exercise helps control weight and is essential for maintaining physical and cardiovascular fitness.[33] It also helps keep cholesterol levels down and reduce the likelihood of diabetes. Lack of physical activity is linked to an increased risk in heart disease for several reasons. A sedentary lifestyle often results in a person becoming overweight or obese because it can be difficult to balance the amount of energy consumed and energy spent (calories are measurements of energy). It can also contribute to the development of diabetes, and 75 percent of those with diabetes die from some sort of heart or blood vessel disease.[34] The immune system responds positively to exercise, and a healthy body provides some additional safety from developing heart disease. While there is not enough information available on how, exactly, a strong immune system may help reduce the risk of heart disease, it seems that plaque buildup in arteries occurs most seriously around inflamed areas. Infection may be one cause of inflammation, and a strong immune system protects the body against infections.

It has been suggested that the cause of death for as many as 250,000 Americans each year is lack of regular physical activity. This is approximately 12 percent of total deaths each year. More frightening is the relative risk of coronary heart disease associated with a lack of exercise. In other words, people who do not exercise regularly have between 50 to 140 percent greater risk of dying from heart disease than a person who exercises adequately. This risk is comparable to that for high cholesterol, high blood pressure, and cigarette smoking.[35]

The American Heart Association's *Heart Disease and Stroke Statistics—2003 Update* presents many findings regarding exercise and related risks for heart disease. Individuals who do not exercise are also more likely to develop other independent risks for heart disease such as high blood pressure and high cholesterol. Less-fit people have a 30 to 50 percent greater risk of developing high blood pressure than those who exercise regularly. The risks of a sedentary lifestyle are prevalent throughout all sectors of American society. Just over half (51.7 percent) of high school students were enrolled in physical education classes in 2001. However, only a third (32.2 percent) attended classes daily. Physical inactivity is more prevalent among women than men, among blacks and Hispanics than whites, among older than younger adults and among the less affluent than the more affluent. And data show that by the age of 16 or 17, 56 percent of black girls and 31 percent of white girls report no habitual physical activity in their leisure time.[36]

The number of people engaging in regular physical activity has leveled off or declined in recent years, after steadily increasing during the 1960s,

1970s, and early 1980s, while the number of obese and overweight is increasing. Since about the early 1990s, only minor changes in leisure time physical activity have occurred.[37] Surveys report that 38 percent of adults (age 18 and older) get no regular exercise; 62 percent get some exercise but not enough and not to a degree of intensity that it protects their hearts. Less than 25 percent get enough exercise to maintain cardiovascular health. Those with lower income levels and less than a twelfth-grade education are more likely to have an inactive lifestyle.[38]

What is enough exercise? This is difficult to measure. It depends on intensity and type of exercise. Recent studies suggest low- to moderate-intensity activities can benefit the heart if done for 30 minutes or more daily. These include walking, climbing stairs, yard work, dancing, and home exercise. Higher-intensity aerobic activities such as running, brisk walking, swimming, and cycling done for at least 30 minutes on most days of the week do more to improve fitness. Several interesting patterns emerged in recent studies about exercise and heart disease risk. The National Academy of Sciences recently upped its suggested amount of daily exercise for maintaining health to an hour each day of the week.[39] Another study found that for older men at least, even though greater amounts of exercise have been shown to have the most benefits in lowering heart disease risk, those whose workouts fall below recommended guidelines but who feel the workouts were vigorous or strenuous also show benefits.[40] Yet a different study showed total physical activity, running, weight training, and walking each reduced coronary heart disease risk, and average exercise intensity was associated with reduced risk independent of the total volume of physical activity.[41] Clearly, the public health concern with lack of exercise is warranted, and the problems related to inactivity are an area that, if addressed successfully, will help continue the progress against heart disease.

## OBESITY, OVERWEIGHT, AND METABOLIC SYNDROME

Obesity affects approximately one in three (more than 61 million) adult Americans, and another 68 million or so are overweight but not obese. Additionally, an estimated 8.8 million young people ages 6 to 19 are overweight or obese. Overweight is judged as a body-mass index (BMI) of 25.0 or greater, and obesity is a BMI of 30.0 or higher. The BMI equals the ratio of weight (in kilograms) to height (in meters squared).[42] For example, a man 5 feet, 10 inches tall (or 1.778 meters, and 3.1613 meters squared) would be overweight if he weighed 174–208 pounds (or 78.9–94.3 kilograms) and would be obese if he weighed 209 pounds or more; a woman 5 feet, 6 inches tall would be overweight if she weighed 155–185 pounds, and would be obese if she weighed 186 pounds or more.

General lack of physical activity and diets based on high-calorie, low-cost foods are major factors in causing obesity and overweight. Obesity and overweight increase heart and blood vessel disease risk because they affect blood lipid levels and LDL cholesterol levels. Obesity substantially raises the risk of hypertension, high cholesterol, asthma, type 2 diabetes, stroke, gallbladder disease, arthritis, osteoarthritis, sleep apnea, respiratory problems, heart disease, and endometrial, breast, prostate, and colon cancers.[43] Chronic diseases associated with obesity, including heart disease and stroke, are the cause of more than two-thirds of all deaths in the United States. The effects of diseases associated with obesity disrupt the daily activities of more than 1 out of every 10 Americans, or approximately 25 million people.[44]

The National Institutes of Health sponsored preventative medicine conferences in 1973 and 1977 that dealt with obesity as a public health problem.[45] Controversy regarding the cause-and-effect relationship between obesity and ill health characterized these conferences, but their focus on these issues emphasizes the importance the medical community has placed for three decades now on the effects of obesity and overweight for overall health. A 1985 National Institutes of Health Consensus Development Conference addressed the health implications of obesity. Providing important national recognition of the seriousness of obesity as a health condition that leads to increased morbidity and mortality, the conference concluded that both prevention and treatment of obesity were medical priorities in the United States. The results of this conference included defining the terms *overweight* and *obesity* as risks to health.

In 1990, the official health goals for Americans for the year 2000 were set forth in the Healthy People 2000 initiative. Among the initiative's stated goals was reducing the prevalence of overweight. In the Healthy People 2010 initiative, the specific goals are to reduce overweight and obesity among adolescents and obesity among adults.[46] Overweight and obesity are among the top 10 leading health indicators, along with physical activity, behind the Healthy People 2010 program.

In 1993, a study concluded that dietary factors and sedentary activity patterns combined account for at least 300,000 adult deaths each year, and that obesity is a key contributor in these deaths.[47] For the next several years, research focused on extreme obesity as a risk factor. The association between extreme obesity and heart failure was shown conclusively earlier, but in 2002, overweight and lesser degrees of obesity as well were strongly and independently linked to increased risk. One study reports the finding of researchers who had followed five thousand participants in the landmark Framingham Heart Study for 15 years. They found that obese women were twice as likely to develop heart failure compared with normal-weight women, and obese men had a 90 percent increased risk. Overweight men and women experience a 34 percent higher risk than normal-weight individuals. With each increase of one in the BMI, a man's risk of heart failure increases 5 percent and a woman's risk increases 7 percent.[48]

The *Heart Disease and Stroke Statistics—2003 Update* from the American Heart Association reported some staggering findings related to obesity and overweight and heart disease. The report estimates that the annual cost of obesity-related diseases in the United States is high, running up to about $100 billion. The annual hospital costs for obese children and adolescents were $127 million during the years 1997 through 1999.[49] Obesity, a major risk factor for cardiovascular disease as well as other chronic diseases, endangers the health of many Americans. In fact, research findings show that obesity, overweight, and diabetes among adult Americans continue to increase in both sexes, all ages, all races, all educational levels, and all smoking levels.[50]

Metabolic syndrome, closely related to overweight and obesity, is another concern of fairly recent development. It is a risk factor for developing diabetes and heart disease as well as increased death from heart disease. Metabolic syndrome is showing up more often in American adults. Also know as "syndrome X," it is defined by the occurrence of three or more of five specific abnormalities associated with increased blood sugar, blood lipids and blood pressure during aging. For men, a waist circumference greater than 40 inches is considered abnormal, and for women, 35 inches. A blood triglyceride level of 150 mg/dL or higher, often linked to high insulin levels, is a second signifying abnormality. A third symptom is a low HDL level, less than 40 mg/dL in men and 50 mg/dL in women. A fourth sign is high blood pressure at or above 130/85. And fifth is a fasting glucose level or 110 mg/dL or higher. Using population numbers from the 2000 census, an estimated 47 million Americans have metabolic syndrome, translating to an age-adjusted prevalence of 23.7 percent of Americans.[51]

## THE TRENDS

The trends observed over the last several decades in areas related to diet, exercise, and heart and blood-vessel disease have not always showed continued progress. The major area where specialists see disturbing trends away from national health goals are the increasing prevalence of overweight and obesity among Americans and of type 2 diabetes, especially with symptoms appearing more often in children and adolescents. The number of overweight Americans increased from 46 percent in 1976–1980 to 55.9 percent in 1988–1994 to 64.5 percent in 1999–2000. Over the same periods, obesity increased from 14.4 percent to 22.9 percent to 30.5 percent, and severe obesity (BMI of 40 or greater) increased from 2.9 percent in 1988–1994 to 4.7 percent in 1999–2000. The increases showed for both men and women in all age groups and for non-Hispanic whites, non-Hispanic blacks, and Mexican Americans. Non-Hispanic black women over age 40 had the highest prevalence of obesity and overweight of all groups, with more than 80 percent overweight and 50 percent obese.[52]

The prevalence of diabetes has also increased significantly, from 4.9 percent in 1990 to 6.5 percent in 1998 to 7.3 percent in 2000 and 7.9 percent in 2001; increases occurred across both sexes, all age ranges, all ethnic groups, and all education levels. Approximately 75 percent of individuals with diabetes die of heart or blood vessel diseases.[53] In 2002, the combined prevalence of diabetes and obesity was almost 3 percent.

Related to the increase in prevalence of overweight, obesity, and diabetes is the observed reversal of trends in daily caloric intake for Americans ages 18 and older. Between 1965 and 1991, total daily calories dropped from 2,049 to 1,807, but by 1996, the average had risen back to 2,000 calories per day.[54] Another observed reversal in nutrition trends is linked to daily intake of dietary fat. From 1965 to 1996, total fat as a proportion of daily calories fell from 39.1 percent to 33.1 percent, and saturated fat declined from 14.4 percent to 11 percent. But looking at just the years 1991 to 1996, Americans ate more calories per day and their daily total fat consumption increased to 74.8 grams, up from 70.9 grams. In 1965, only 1.9 percent of fat intake came from pizza, Mexican food, Chinese food, hamburgers, French fries, and cheeseburgers. In 1994–1996, these six foods accounted for 10.8 percent of total fat in the diet.[55]

Not all the trends are negative. The percentage of adults ages 29 to 74 with high blood cholesterol (greater than 240 mg/dL) decreased from 32 percent in 1960–1962 to 19 percent in 1988–1994. Mean blood cholesterol levels of adults 18 and older dropped from 220 in the early 1960s to 203 in the mid-1990s. The amount of calories in the diet from fat and from saturated fat also dropped, from 36 percent to 34 percent and from 13 percent to 12 percent, respectively, from 1976–1980 to 1988–1994.[56] The proportion of fat calories from major sources of saturated fat, including beef, dairy products (especially whole milk), and eggs, as well as from pork, fell from about half in 1965 to about one-third by 1994–1996. Meanwhile, the percentage of calories from poultry and fruits and vegetables rose substantially, and the percentage of adults who ate fruits and vegetables at least five times a day increased between 1990 and 1996.[57] These trends show overall improvements, and although in some cases the observable improvement is only a small percentage, the number of lives saved is unarguably significant.

A review of more than five decades of overall progress against heart disease indicates both positive and negative trends. There is positive proof that many Americans are changing their lifestyles to improve their health. Negative progress or inadequate change shows that many Americans are moving away from set targets for improving health despite advances in knowledge and treatment of heart and blood vessel disease. The poor performance in the areas of overweight, obesity, and diabetes indicates focal areas for future efforts against heart disease, while the dietary improvements may have reached a plateau. Considering all the available information about heart disease and the risk factors associated with diet and exercise, the question emerges: Do Americans care enough about their health to make what may be difficult changes to their lifestyles?

## CLOSING REMARKS

The remarkable progress against heart disease that was evident throughout the second half of the twentieth century was in large part the result of better understanding of how the body's metabolic processes work and applying the knowledge of risk factors to dietary behavior. Further progress in successfully treating and preventing heart disease can be made through changes in diet and physical activity. However, the initial, more rapid stages of progress by these means appear to have come to a close, and in the future, the changes Americans may have to make to reduce their risk for heart disease could be difficult. Instead of seeing steps to take in the future as "sacrifices," Americans must remember that improving their health improves their quality of life, and one of America's core values is that hard work leads to positive results. The cost to Americans of poor diet, sedentary lifestyle, and obesity is astounding. More than $33 billion in medical costs and $9 billion in lost productivity due to heart disease, cancer, stroke, and diabetes are attributed to diet. The cost of diseases including but not limited to heart disease and diabetes related to a sedentary lifestyle is an estimated $76 billion each year. And treatment of heart disease related to obesity and overweight among U.S. adults in the most recent year data has been compiled (1996) was $31 billion.[58] Past improvements in the health of Americans will continue to save money, improve productivity, and ensure a more satisfying life only if Americans do more to eat a more nutritious diet, exercise more regularly, and manage the consumption of calories.

# CHAPTER 8

# Stress and Psychological Factors

On Saturday, June 22, 2002, Major League Baseball player Darryl Kile was scheduled to start as pitcher for the St. Louis Cardinals in a game against the Chicago Cubs. When he failed to show up at the clubhouse before the game, team officials contacted the hotel where the players were staying and asked the management to check on the pitcher. Hotel security went to his room, saw the door with a "Do Not Disturb" sign hanging from the handle, and forced their way into the room. There they found the young pitcher dead, apparently having died during his sleep of a heart attack. An autopsy later showed blockages of 80 to 90 percent in his coronary arteries.

Kile, age 33, was an admired and well-liked veteran pitcher who had played for the Houston Astros and Colorado Rockies before going to the St. Louis Cardinals. He had a great sense of humor, according to those who knew him, and was active off the field. In the off-season, he was known as an excellent golfer, hitting the links for charity tournaments and for fun. The father of three, he was seemingly healthy. As a professional athlete, he underwent routine physical exams, none of which had shown anything out of the ordinary.

Kile was one of the top pitchers in the game. In 1993, he accomplished the rare feat of throwing a no-hitter. In 1997, he won 19 games, and in 2000, he won 20 games, both impressive years. During his major league career of 11-plus seasons, he finished twice in the top five for the Cy Young award, the yearly honor that goes to the best pitcher in each league, and was a three-time All-Star.

Achieving so much success over several long and grueling seasons, Kile was outwardly healthy and in shape. He had passed his yearly preseason physical, which included an ECG and blood tests—they had shown nothing irregular. He was active, had a supportive and caring family and social network, and had never complained of chest pain or other symptoms that may have indicated heart disease. In hindsight, however, it is easy to see at least a couple of signs that suggest Kile was at increased risk for heart disease. His father died at age 44 from a heart attack—the genetic risk factor. He also may have been at risk from stress, a less well established and understood risk.

Kile worked and lived in an extremely competitive, stressful environment. The life of a Major League Baseball player includes not only the physical and psychological demands of each game but the stress of traveling regularly, of being away from family, and of never knowing for sure how long one will be with any team. Kile had played in Houston, Denver, and St. Louis during his career. Players also experience a lot of pressure from fans, sponsors, management, and the media. In his early days playing for Houston, the team was not winning and the fans often booed the team and players while the media ridiculed their effort. These and other stress factors may have played a role in the development of Kile's atherosclerosis.

Unfortunately, sudden deaths such as Darryl Kile's are not rare. Approximately 250,000 people die each year of heart attacks without showing symptoms, and in 90 percent of sudden deaths in adults, atherosclerosis has narrowed at least two of the major coronary arteries. On the one hand, because of his father's death, Kile could have been a candidate for more intensive heart exams. On the other hand, an outwardly healthy and active person without obvious symptoms might easily be taken as an unlikely candidate for premature heart disease. There are tests that could have shown his short-term risk, a CT coronary calcification exam for example, but the need for such a test only became apparent after his death.[1]

## WHAT IS STRESS AND HOW DOES IT AFFECT THE HEART?

Stress exhibits itself in many forms, from anger and hostility toward another person or oneself to perspiration and heavy breathing after exercise. Stress is not "bad" in and of itself. In fact, were it not for stress, human beings would have a difficult time surviving, and our earliest ancestors probably would have died out long before today's humans evolved. Stress is an essential physical, psychological, and emotional response to certain situations. It helps the body stay alive in difficult moments. At the same time, the effects of chronic stress can devastate the body over time. Stress, while necessary, is not healthy. Information gathered over the past several years makes it increasingly clear that the amount of stress one experiences and how one deals with it over a lifetime can seriously affect the heart.

A person who perceives danger will often notice telltale signs of stress—breathlessness, an acute sense of awareness, and a pounding heart. Most of what happens in the body during stress goes unnoticed; nonetheless, these signals indicate that the body is prepared to defend itself, either by fighting or by fleeing. The internal response to stress improves the body's reflexes, strength, agility, and ability to cool itself with perspiration. One's body remains in this state of preparedness until the danger subsides. When the threat has passed, the body relaxes and slowly returns to normal. Over time, chronic stress and other stress-related factors can impair the body's ability to calm down.

Most events that cause stress on a daily basis in today's world are not life threatening, nor do they require one to fight or run away. Often they are relatively minor details blown out of proportion, like a burst of anger at a person driving slow in the fast lane or an argument caused by an unpleasant exchange with a coworker. At other times, when severe pressure to meet expectations and routine deadlines at work or a festering conflict with a spouse is present, the details may not be minor, but one's immediate survival is not at stake. Or is it?

Humans evolved physiologically to deal with high-risk, short-duration stress—fight or flight—not the low-risk, long-duration stress people regularly face today. People under stress are not in a physically healthy condition, and people who thrive in high-pressure, busy environments are able to do so without experiencing (or by tempering) their natural stress response. The physiological responses that mark stress are high blood pressure, elevated heart rate, increased production of blood-clotting agents, and raised metabolic rate. This exhausts the body and over the long haul can result in overexertion of the heart. The World Health Organization's *World Health Report 2002* identified high blood pressure as the second most important cause of death and disability in developed countries, second only to tobacco.[2]

Both physiological and psychology effects of stress can cause harm. The physiological effects—those biological and chemical effects observed in the body—are reasonably well established and understood. Measuring the psychological effects of stress presents certain difficulties, especially because people respond in unique ways to a given set of circumstances, and the relationship between emotions and physical processes are hard to quantify. The psychological profiles and questionnaires used to determine how a person feels are highly subjective. Based on self-reporting, the most effective questionnaires require the interviewer to interpret *how* a person responds to each question as well as what the person says.

Because of the limited amount of clinical and statistical information available, some debate exists over how to deal with the issue of stress-related heart disease. While the association between stress and heart disease is established, the evidence collected so far is considered inadequate for treating it in the same way as other primary risk factors. There are some in the United States, researcher and author Dr. Meyer Friedman for one, who go so far as to claim that Type A behavior (a psychosocial factor linked to personality and behavior) may be the single most important risk factor for heart disease and may actually cause some of the primary risk factors such as high cholesterol, smoking, and type 2 diabetes associated with heart disease.[3] This view has not gained wide acceptance but has raised a whole new set of issues about preventing and treating heart disease. While full understanding is unlikely to come any time soon, stress certainly seems to compound the risk of heart disease when present with other primary risk factors such as smoking, high cholesterol, obesity, lack of exercise, hypertension, diabetes, or genetic predisposition. This compounding effect can be seen by comparing the normal heart rate of someone smoking cigarettes with a smoker under stress. Smoking raises a person's heartbeat on average 14 beats per minute, but when combined with stress, it rises to 38 beats per minute.[4]

---

## TYPE A VERSUS TYPE B BEHAVIOR

Presidents Kennedy and Johnson were Type A personalities, while Presidents Ford and Reagan were Type B personalities. The difference has nothing to do with their political party or success as a leader, and each revealed a unique individual personality while in office. So how do Type A and Type B behavior differ? How do the differences show up in everyday life? Confusion seems common. At one time, it became faddish to label friends and acquaintances as Type A or Type B. Yet, some people treat their Type A behavior as a badge of their accomplishment and a trait to take pride in, while others view it as a symptom of underlying insecurity and unhappiness. Here is a brief guide to the key characteristics of each.[5]

In general terms, Type A behavior is "above all a continuous struggle, an unremitting attempt to accomplish more and more things or participate in more and more events in less and less time, frequently in the face of opposition—real or imagined—from other persons." Type A behavior ultimately stems from a sense of insecurity and lack of self-esteem but shows up in two major traits. One trait is a sense of time urgency or "hurry sickness." Those with the trait accelerate the pace at which they think, plan, and act in daily life, eventually reaching the point of becoming obsessed with efficiency and speed. Another trait is free-floating hostility toward people, things, and the world in general that slow their pace or obstruct their progress. In contrast, Type B behavior is defined in terms of the absence of these behavioral traits and the underlying struggle of daily life.

Persons with Type A behavior are often told by friends and loved ones to slow down and enjoy life, but they seldom heed this advice. They talk fast, walk fast, eat fast, and hate (much more than most) to wait in lines, be stuck in traffic, listen to someone talk leisurely, and spend time alone with nothing to do. Relaxing is hard and usually involves competitive sports, work-related socializing, or some sort of activity that involves accomplishment. Typically, moving quickly isn't fast enough by itself, so Type A persons try to do several things at once. To gain more time, they brush their teeth and plan for the day at the same time, they read work-related papers while eating, they dictate letters or make business calls while driving, they write memos while on the phone, and they watch TV and read at the same time. They cite statistics and numbers to convey information quickly rather than speak in terms of images and metaphors, and they want speed and action in entertainment rather than beauty and art. They work best on deadlines, and impose deadlines on themselves if outside ones don't exist. In short, packing as many activities as possible into as short a time as possible seems to be the major goal.

In the face of the effort to get so many things done so quickly, people and external events invariably obstruct this effort. The response of those with Type A behavior is aggression and hostility. The behavior shows in excessive anger over petty annoyances: the mistakes of other drivers, the slowness and mistakes of clerks in stores or government offices, loud and sometimes impolite teenagers, opposing political views and beliefs, and the actions of competitors at work and play. It's easy for anyone to find things to be annoyed by, but for the Type A personality these annoyances provoke anger, hostility, and aggressiveness.

Type B behavior, in contrast, involves patience, less attention to the passage of time, and a long-term perspective on one's goals. Those with Type B behavior meet deadlines, accomplish goals, and move forward in their life, but without the frenzy of those with Type A behavior. They are more prone to delegate to others and accept the occasional imperfections of coworkers, subordinates, and family members. They tend to overlook annoyances without turning daily irritations into major aggravations and can correct problems they face without becoming filled with anger. They recognize their shortcomings and strengths, but without exaggerating the former and minimizing the latter. They do one thing at a time with the goal of doing it with both enjoyment and care. While Type A persons tend to impress initially with their energy, Type B persons tend to impress with their security and tranquility.

Both behavior types have characteristics that people admire, but one characteristic makes Type A behavior less desirable than Type B behavior: It is associated with heart disease and early death.

## WHAT IS A STRESS RESPONSE?

A stress response involves a person's reaction to physical, chemical, emotional, or environmental factors. Mental tension and physical effort both result in stress. Mounting evidence suggests a relationship between psychosocial and environmental factors and cardiovascular risk, including job strain, social isolation, and personality traits. Exactly how stress affects heart risk is unknown, although a large body of evidence sheds light on the relationship. Other known primary risk factors for heart disease, such as high cholesterol and high blood pressure, have been shown to be associated with stress. Stress is also linked to an increased tendency to smoke, gain weight, and decrease physical activity. Despite the implications of the existence of such links, the American Heart Association says more evidence is needed to make specific recommendations about stress-management to reduce heart risk.[6]

People experience stress every day as a part of life, and mostly, they deal with it as it arises. How they handle it depends on the person—something causing an extreme stress response in one person may result in a mild response or none at all in another. For instance, walking through Times Square in New York City along sidewalks congested with people, the smell of exhaust, and the constant bombardment of lights, noise, and movement is a potentially stressful situation. For a New Yorker who is accustomed to the hustle and bustle of the city, the walk may seem hardly extraordinary and just a part of living in the city. For a first-time visitor to the city, the experience may cause a rising heartbeat, a feeling of physical or psychological discomfort, and perhaps the perception of a threat from somewhere among all the commotion. Another visitor with prior experience in the city may feel many of the same emotions as the first-time visitor, except instead of feeling threatened, that person may feel comfortable or even elated by the experience of seeing it all again. All three types of people experience the same environmental causes of stress (stressors) from walking through the mayhem of Times Square, yet their reactions and therefore their stress responses are different. One's stress response is based at least in part by survival instincts from the evolutionary past. Experienced on irregular occasions, there is little or nothing to worry about from an extreme stress response. If extreme stress becomes chronic, however, then a person's health and well-being are at risk, specifically, their heart and blood vessels.

Because people respond to stressful situations in a number of ways depending on their personality, the gravity of the situation, and other factors, it is difficult to generalize situations and the stress responses they will provoke. Still, in most stressful situations, whether caused by physical or emotional distress, the body behaves according to an established physiological process that has been ingrained in human biology. One theory of how stress directly affects the heart and the rest of the body is centered on a hormonal system known as the hypothalamic-pituitary-adrenal (HPA) axis. The HPA axis corresponds to a highly ordered process whereby, in response to stress, the nervous system triggers the release of several hormones throughout the body. First, a section of the brain called the hypothalamus releases what is known as corticotrophin-releasing hormone (CRH). Next, CRH signals the pituitary gland, which lays just beneath the brain, to release adrenocorticotropin (ACTH), another hormone. This then signals the adrenal glands (located near the kidneys) to release numerous other hormones. Three of these are epinephrine (adrenaline), norepinephrine (noradrenaline), and cortisol. Together, these enable the body to defend itself from attack. Epinephrine and norepinephrine increase the blood pressure and heart rate, divert blood flow to the muscles, and speed reaction time. Cortisol releases glucose (sugar) reserves, which the muscles and brain use as energy. This process also affects other systems throughout the body that can affect the heart, notably the autonomic nervous system.[7]

The autonomic nervous system helps people adjust to changes in their environment by regulating and modifying how the body functions in response to stress. The sympathetic and parasympathetic nervous systems together make up the autonomic nervous system. The sympathetic nervous system causes excitement or arousal by quickening blood-vessel contractions, slowing intestinal ones, and increasing the heartbeat to prepare the body for exertion, emotional stress, and extreme cold. The sympathetic nervous system activates other physiological responses to help the body survive. It can make the heart pump more blood to the brain, muscles, and surface of the skin, and it can speed up and deepen breathing. It can also elevate blood-sugar and fatty acid levels, slow down digestion, cause skin perspiration, and dilate the pupils to let in additional light, as well as control orgasm during sexual arousal. The parasympathetic nervous system slows many bodily functions and calms or relaxes a person. When the sympathetic and parasympathetic nervous systems are balanced, the autonomic nervous system helps regulate the size of blood vessels and blood pressure, the heart's electrical ability and contractions, and the diameter of the bronchus and amount of air reaching the lungs. An imbalance of the autonomic nervous system caused by chronic or acute stress may promote the development of atherosclerosis and can trigger lethal arrhythmias.[8] An overly strong sympathetic nervous system and a weak parasympathetic nervous system can result in a number of other risk-increasing developments: increased heart rate, increased levels of free fatty acids and cholesterol in the blood, increased clumping of platelets, and decreased immune system functioning.[9]

The HPA axis also affects parts of the brain responsible for controlling motivation and mood, fear in response to danger, memory formation, and vital functions including body temperature, appetite suppression, and pain control. When the body faces danger, the HPA axis activates a stress response that shuts off the hormonal systems that regulate growth, reproduction, metabolism, and immunity and redirects all available resources to those functions most vital for survival. Each individual's stress response is unique because of biological differences in the genes that control the HPA axis and because the functioning of the HPA axis can be altered by experiences of extreme stress at any point in the life cycle from womb to adulthood.[10] For example, individuals of all types who live in a war-ravaged area may develop an extremely sensitive stress response after facing years of repeated stress.

Stress also causes the body to release free fatty acids and glucose into the blood stream, providing energy to sustain or flee from the threat of attack. In a real life-or-death situation, these calories are likely to be used in the physical fight for survival. Because most stressful situations today are not life-or-death conflicts—in fact, they often involve work, family, or other parts of the daily routine—an aggressive physical response is in most cases no longer required. Without physical exertion, the extra free fatty acids and glucose in the blood can contribute to the buildup of materials on vessel walls that block or constrict blood flow. If repeated often over time, this process can elevate cholesterol levels and result in chronic hypertension, both of which are associated with increased risk of heart disease.[11]

Yet another response to stress, particularly that caused by injury, manifests itself in the form of the body producing and releasing additional blood-clotting agents. These blood-clotting particles may attach themselves to any lesion or scratch in the arteries. Combined with cholesterol and other materials, the clots tend to block the flow of blood through the artery to the heart. Stress causes the heart to work extra hard, and this overexertion weakens the heart, making it more susceptible to damage and less able to deal with some of the problems associated with heart disease.

## HEART DISEASE MORTALITY AND PSYCHOSOCIAL FACTORS

Acute and chronic stress affect the body in ways that regular, mild, daily stress does not. Five types of psychosocial stress are linked to heart disease: depression, anxiety, anger or hostility, social isolation, and chronic life stress. At least some of the links between psychological stress and heart disease appear to result from an overactive sympathetic nervous system, which may accelerate the development of atherosclerosis. An elevated heart rate and blood pressure characterize the exaggerated response to stress. Psychosocial stress factors often appear together, sharing many underlying roots. Similarly, established risk factors for heart disease such as obesity, poor diet, and lack of exercise also tend to occur together in the same individual because they stem from similar behavioral patterns. For individuals who suffer from one or more sources of psychosocial stress, the resulting risk for a cardiac event equals that associated with factors such as hypertension and high levels of cholesterol.[12]

The first studies to examine how emotions and feelings affect the heart began in the 1950s. Out of these studies came the term *Type A personality*. Hostility, a combination of cynicism, anger, and aggression, was later shown to be a significant predictor of heart disease, while the other elements of Type A behavior—ambition, impatience, time urgency, competitiveness, and personal work and achievement drive—did not predict heart disease.[13] Comparative research on mortality rates among people treated for major depression and the general population began in the 1970s, with 9 of 10 studies agreeing that depressed people die from coronary heart disease more often than nondepressed people.[14] The studies identified the existence of the relationship, yet they shed little light on how causes or treatments might affect outcome. In early studies, the portion of observed risk attributable to other risk factors such as smoking, heavy drinking, and inactivity was not examined. Later, investigators found a strong association between depression and cigarette smoking. The first study to control for smoking appeared in 1993, and the relation between depression and mortality persisted. It also showed a relation between depression and the development of ischemic heart disease.

During the mid-1990s, several community surveys followed populations that were initially free of heart disease. Of these studies, most found an increased risk of ischemic heart disease among those individuals who suffered depression. Other studies followed subjects who had preexisting heart disease, and among these results, depression was linked with a worse outcome. One of these studies concluded that patients who were depressed after a heart attack were 3.5 times more likely to die compared with depression-free individuals.[15] During the first two decades or so of research, investigators raised many questions about the psychosocial risk factors for heart disease, especially depression and personality type, and they pinpointed a broad range of areas for future research. Yet, in terms of observable results, progress in managing the negative effects of stress on the heart and improving mortality was limited or nonexistent. Researchers still needed to define the exact mechanisms by which risk increased and develop proven strategies for beating the problem.

In 2000, investigators found that intense physical activities and mental activities increase the likelihood of cardiac ischemia (where blood flow and oxygen are unable to get to the heart), and that anger is a major trigger of ischemia, with sadness, frustration, and tension also possible triggers. Tests showed that mental stressors can trigger ischemia in 40 to 70 percent of patients with heart disease.[16] In 2002, researchers found a concrete connection between mental or emotional stress and increased risk of heart disease. Using ultrasound to observe blood vessels in individuals before a 3-minute stress test and then again 10 minutes after, researchers found the inner layer of blood vessel had constricted while blood pressure and heart rates had increased. Reporting their findings, the researchers concluded that sudden mental anguish (one form of stress) makes blood vessels less able to respond to changes in blood flow. It also can induce endothelial dysfunction, a condition whereby the blood vessels are unable to dilate properly, increasing risk of developing atherosclerosis.[17]

Of the most recent studies of the relationship between stress and heart trouble, some stand out for what they reveal about potential differences between men and women. One examination of Japanese men and women found that women who reported high levels of mental stress had 2.28 times the risk of coronary heart disease and 1.64 times the risk of any heart-related death compared with women who reported low stress levels. The high-stress women were on average five years younger, thinner, and more educated, but also less physically active and more likely to have a history of hypertension or diabetes than those reporting low stress. They also smoked more and were more likely to work full-time. Researchers also found these high-stress women were more likely to be angry, to be in a hurry, to feel hopeless, and to feel unfulfilled. In the same study, men reporting medium to high levels of stress had a risk of heart attack 1.74 times compared with men who experienced low stress.[18]

Another study found women were more likely to suffer sudden cardiac arrest triggered by psychosocial stress than by physical exercise. For men, physical exercise was the more common trigger. Researchers hypothesized that the release of adrenaline triggered by physical exertion or by emotional distress was the cause of the heart attack.[19] As the evidence mounts that stress can damage the heart and even cause death, the need for more research into how to intervene successfully and reduce this danger becomes increasingly obvious. Although our understanding is incomplete, what follows is a brief look at some of the information researchers have gathered about these various risks.

### Depression and Anxiety

Depressive symptoms pose an independent risk for onset of coronary heart disease, with the risk being 1.64 times higher than for those without depressive symptoms.[20] A focus of much recent research is the onset of depression after a coronary heart event. Symptoms of depression appear within a week after a heart attack in up to half the patients studied. Moreover, several studies indicate that heart disease can also follow depression.[21] The established facts show that people with heart disease are more likely to have depression than healthy people; in fact, the overall American adult population experiences depression in any given year at a ratio of about 1 in 20, while 1 in 3 survivors of heart attacks showed signs of depression. As many as one in five individuals exhibit signs of clinical (severe) depression after suffering a heart disease. Unfortunately, despite the risks for a worse prognosis and even death, depression is rarely treated in heart patients.[22] How much the severity and duration of depressive symptoms and disorders affects coronary risk remains to be determined. Although the combination of depression and heart disease is associated with increased sickness and death, it remains unclear whether treating depression actually improves the prognosis for heart disease. In the past, many medications used to treat depression had complicating side effects on heart disease. More recent antidepression medications, particularly selective serotonin reuptake inhibitors such as Prozac and Zoloft, do not have the same negative impact on the heart as earlier drugs.[23]

By the mid-1990s, researchers had found that depressed patients were more likely to die than those not depressed. Investigators in Montreal found high levels of sadness and depression in heart patients that increased their risk of death in the next 18 months by eight times. Anxiety and anger each tripled the risk.[24] A simultaneous study in Baltimore, Maryland, assessed more than 1,500 people who initially did not have heart disease and found that those with a history of depression had four times the number of heart attacks over the next 14 years compared with those without depression.[25]

Why do people with depression seem more prone to developing heart problems and to die sooner than those who are not depressed? Some forms of severe depression result in a response called "learned helplessness," which is characterized by several symptoms linked to increased heart risk—anxiety, rapid heartbeat, high blood pressure, and high cholesterol and triglyceride levels. People with learned helplessness also tend to produce high levels of CRH (the hormone that triggers stress response) and cortisol. Anxiety disorder and poorly controlled diabetes are conditions associated with high levels of CRH and cortisol, and cortisol can increase appetite and lead to weight gain. As a result, persistent high levels of these hormones can have a negative effect on heart risk.[26] In addition, depressed heart patients find it more difficult to take medication and follow their doctors' directions on modifying behavior and lifestyle. They thus do less well in reducing their risk of subsequent heart attacks after an initial heart attack.[27]

These findings raise important questions about who might benefit most from treatment of psychosocial stressors, although it remains to be seen if there is an effective way of treating depression and anxiety in heart patients. With more researchers now interested in studying these problems, one can anticipate additional progress against heart disease. Because depression may increase coronary risk by 50 to 60 percent for patients with minor depression compared with nondepressed patients, and because major depression carries a risk more than twice as high, many people may potentially benefit from new treatments.[28] However, a recent study suggests that only those heart attack patients with mild depression showed benefits for cardiac mortality with improvement in their depression symptoms. For those with severe depression after their heart event, treating their depression may not effectively improve their risk.[29]

### Anger and Hostility

How people respond to psychological and social stress strongly relates to the effects of stress on the heart. The authors of the book *Anger Kills* wrote the following about some of the main causes of stress, the everyday anger, annoyance, and irritation many people feel: "[G]etting angry is like taking a small dose of some slow-acting poison—arsenic, for example— every day of your life. . . . Anger is a toxin to your body."[30] Anger is just one manifestation of how a person deals with stress, and it is not alone in damaging one's health. People also deal with stress in other ways that can damage their heart and their overall health—by overeating, by smoking, by consuming too much alcohol, and by failing to exercise. These behaviors alone present serious risks to the heart, but combined with stress they may become even more dangerous.

Chronically angry men, for example, have a higher risk for heart disease than men who get angry less. Yet, a recent study that examined more than 23,000 men over two years found those with moderate expressions of anger had about half the risk of nonfatal heart attacks compared with those who do not express their anger. The participants were more educated, had reached older ages, came from a higher socioeconomic status, and had lower anger levels than the average population. Still, the findings indicate that those who bury their anger within instead of expressing it increase their risk for coronary heart disease.[31]

Type A personality (also called coronary-prone behavior pattern) defines a cluster of behaviors that can harm the heart. As described earlier, one trait associated with Type A personality is hostility, which appears to have the strongest association with the development and progression of heart disease. In general, Type A people have been found to produce more epinephrine and norepinephrine (hormones that prepare the body to deal with stress and struggle) and to have higher levels of the hormone circulating through their blood stream than Type B (non–Type A) individuals.[32] These hormones increase the heart rate, demand for oxygen by the heart muscle, and strain on the cardiovascular system.

Hostile people are at risk not only from their outlook and their hypersensitive stress response (fight or flight preparation), but also because they are more likely to be smokers, to drink more alcohol, and to consume more calories. Hostility appears higher among individuals who have low socioeconomic status, are nonwhites, and face other risk factors.[33] Interestingly, hostile people react differently than nonhostile people to anger and irritation—as anger increases, so does their heart rate, blood pressure, blood flow to muscles, and amount of stress hormones released. In contrast, nonhostile people, who avoid anger rather than hide or express it, show little association between hostile emotions and physiologic reactivity. Hostile people also tend to possess a weak parasympathetic nervous system (the system responsible for calming and slowing the heart rate) and a weak immune system. Hostile people may suffer from lower levels of brain serotonin, which could explain why they react to situations differently than nonhostile people. Raising brain serotonin has been shown both in animals and in humans to decrease appetite and help weight loss, where decreasing it leads subjects to eat more and gain weight.[34] On a side note, although Type A people are more likely than others to have a heart attack, some research suggests the more easygoing Type B person is more likely than the Type A person to die after heart disease is diagnosed, possibly because Type A personalities are likely to take recovery as a personal challenge and work harder on rehabilitation.[35]

Much of the work done on heart disease focuses on older individuals because age increases heart risk. However, the impact of many risk factors including hostility, smoking, and high cholesterol becomes less harmful as age increases. Recently, investigators have looked more specifically at the effects of a lifetime of certain types of behavior and personality traits on coronary heart risk. Anger and hostility appear to predispose young people to several conditions that increase their heart risk prematurely. In young men, high levels of anger caused by stress increase risk of premature heart disease and heart attack. In young adults, hostility has been associated with coronary artery calcification, which is a marker of atherosclerosis.[36]

Optimism, in contrast to anger and hostility, has been associated with decreased risk. Optimists appear to have greater survival rates after a diagnosis of heart disease than pessimists, with 12 percent of pessimists dying within a year compared with only 5 percent of optimists. A patient's outlook, more than severity of condition, predicted a better prognosis. Pessimism appeared to be a greater risk to recovery than depression.[37]

---

## FIVE STEPS TO MANAGING STRESS

*Step 1: Recognize the stress.* Early warning signals of stress include physical signs such as rapid heartbeat, muscle tension, and upset stomach; mental signs such as feelings of worry or distraction; emotional signs such as irritability, anxiety, and temporary depression; and behavioral signs such as temper outbursts, social withdrawal, accident proneness, and substance abuse.

*Step 2: Accept responsibility for responding to stress.* Accepting responsibility for confronting stress empowers a person to deal with the source of the stress, whether it is work, marital problems, or something else. This does not mean blaming oneself for stress but understanding that stress is manageable.

*Step 3: Find the source(s) of stress.* Locate the source of stress, the stressor, whether it is an infrequent major life event (marriage or job loss) or an ongoing, daily strain (an unsatisfying job, commuting in traffic, or nagging debt). Chronic worriers invent the sources of their stress. Then decide if the source of stress is something that can be "fixed." If so, take the steps to improve it.

*Step 4: Examine the beliefs and attitudes that may be associated with stress.* Stress is more complicated than just what happens to a person—how one deals with what happens is more important. Stress is caused in large part by whether a person believes an event or situation is stressful. In other words, because events and situations are themselves neutral, dealing with them in an effective way, such as enjoying the music on the radio when caught in traffic instead of obsessing on it as wasted time, can manage or neutralize the amount of stress they cause.

*Step 5: Employ stress reduction techniques and activities.* Try talking about the problem to a trusted friend, exercising, doing a relaxation technique such as controlled breathing or visualization, getting a massage, taking a warm bath, meditating, spending time on a physically demanding hobby, or seeking out something that will cause laughter.[38]

## Social Isolation and Lack of Social Support

The harm of social isolation and lack of social support is apparent in considering the benefits of the opposite situation. People with a strong network of social support composed of friends, family, or other people to confide in and who live less-solitary lives have better prognoses after heart events than those who do not have close personal ties with others. The most recent Health Survey for England found that men are more likely than women to report lack of social support, by 16 percent to 11 percent. It also found those with higher incomes reported more social support than those with lower incomes.[39] The sense of relief and self-esteem that comes from sharing one's troubles offers a reason to fight hard for recovery. Having others who care often can serve as an essential component of heart rehabilitation.

Social support appears to predict, more than anything else, if and for how long a person will live after a heart event. People who suffer congestive heart failure tend to experience moderate depression in the aftermath, yet higher levels of social support and more positive outlook have a positive impact on prognosis.[40] Investigators recently found that while depression after a heart attack is a predictor of one-year cardiac mortality and social support is not directly related to survival, very high levels of support appear to indirectly lower the negative impact of depression on mortality. High levels of support predict improvements in depression in the first year after a heart attack in depressed patients and long-term chance of survival may improve.[41] By contrast, those who had already experienced one heart attack and who lived alone were at double the risk for recurrent heart attack or death. Moreover, unmarried individuals with heart disease were more likely to die from heart related causes within five years.[42] This psychosocial factor, less conclusively linked to heart disease than others, remains an extremely important factor to consider in relation to heart disease. Helping people with cardiac rehabilitation may be as important for continued progress against heart disease as prevention or intervention.

## Chronic Life Stress

Chronic life stress is something of a catchall category. More important than what causes the stress is its duration. Short periods of difficulty due to a major deadline at work, a marriage, a divorce, or any other irregular cause of stress can trigger a heart event, but chronic life stress relates to those things day in and day out that people face. Chronic stress plays a significant role in speeding up the development of atherosclerosis and acute stress can trigger cardiac events.[43] A long commute, prolonged unhappiness in a relationship, and work tasks that are repetitive and not enjoyable are examples of chronic stress. One element of chronic stress in the workplace occurs when employees feel that they lack control over daily activities. Chronic job-related stress affects both men and women. The British government has acknowledged that "working in jobs which make very high demands, or in which people have little or no control, increases the risk of [heart disease] and premature death."[44]

The damage caused by chronic stress resembles that caused by Type A behavior—it results from a kind of long-term, overactive stress response. Individuals under chronic stress are more likely to have an overactive HPA axis and suffer from depression. Depressed people have impaired ability to regulate their stress response, which causes constant anxiety and overreaction to stimulation. As a result of chronic stress, cortisol may be produced more or less continuously, increasing appetite, leading to weight gain, and resulting in other complications that increase heart risk.[45]

Researchers found that New York City traffic cops, presumably with high-stress jobs, showed lower blood pressure during stressful moments on the job when they reported having social support from their work supervisors. This finding indicates that perceived social support in the workplace may affect the amount of work-related strain placed on the heart.[46] City life in general also appears linked to increased psychosocial stress. Men living in inner London were twice as likely as men living elsewhere in England to have high scores on a health questionnaire designed to evaluate levels of stress, anxiety, and happiness; for women living in London, the observed risk of having high scores increased by 25 percent compared with those living elsewhere.[47]

Long-term marital stress also can aggravate heart conditions. In women aged 30 to 65 with heart disease and married or cohabiting with a male partner, marital stress is associated with an increase of almost three times in the risk for recurrent heart events, even after adjusting for other causes of heart disease. Among working women, however, work stress did not significantly predict recurrent coronary events.[48] Among men, both work stress and marital stress predict increased risk for mortality. Those reporting more than three work stressors faced risks of death 25 percent higher than those with no stressors; and those who are divorced faced risks 37 percent higher than those who remained married.[49]

## REDUCE STRESS AND PROTECT THE HEART?

Researchers have not yet compiled enough evidence to be certain that reducing stress will lower the risk of heart disease, but studies certainly suggest that less hostility and anger and more social ties can improve one's health. Certainly, such proactive measures will not harm one's health. There are, however, certain strategies that doctors often recommend during recovery for heart patients. People who have suffered heart failure should make time during each day to rest so that their hearts can pump blood more easily. This helps to keep them from overexerting themselves and makes coping with tiredness from sleep interruption (a common symptom) less difficult. Rest also helps all people manage stress better. It can help lower blood pressure and prevent overeating, smoking, and excessive drinking. Regular exercise is another way of reducing stress. Older adults suffering from major depression who participated in an exercise program showed similar improvements to those on antidepressants.[50] Exercise is protective against heart risk as well, so one can hope that if more Americans exercise regularly, the number of people with heart disease linked to depression can be reduced.

Dr. Dean Ornish, author of a best-selling book on reversing heart disease, has found that patients who receive a comprehensive cardiac treatment program that supplements routine cardiology care with restrictions on dietary fat consumption, exercise, yoga, and group support sessions show actual shrinkage of coronary lesions and improved heart function without medication.[51] He believes that through the social support element of his program, patients improve their ability to cope effectively with stress, and this is a key reason why his program is so successful. Other studies have also shown techniques such as meditation, relaxation training, stress management, group support, and cognitive therapy for depression can help reduce psychological distress as well as lower blood pressure, heart rate, and cholesterol levels. These therapies apparently help lower mortality rates and recurrence rates during the first couple of years following a coronary event.[52] However, not all studies have found a relationship between reduced risk and psychosocial treatment.

## FINAL REMARKS

Stress affects a person's physical and psychosocial well-being because of the physiological and emotional responses. Inadequate social support, work stress, marital stress, depression, anxiety, and Type A behavior are all significantly associated with an increased risk of heart disease.[53] Yet it is difficult to measure the effects of stress on heart health because how people perceive the world around them is often the factor most indicative of increased risk. As long as the scientific relationship between psychosocial stress and the development of heart disease remains unclear, any progress in treating heart disease by treating psychosocial factors will remain limited. Mounting evidence that depression, anxiety, lack of social support, hostility, and other related factors increase risk for heart disease and worse prognosis should lead to more investigation into this relatively understudied area. Knowing that psychosocial factors increase risk without knowing the precise mechanisms that cause increased risk puts medical professionals in the difficult position of uncertainty about treating these factors.

There is optimism that stress and related psychosocial factors may be areas for which future investigation will turn up results that will lead to additional progress in lowering the prevalence of heart disease among the general population and better the prognosis for those who have already been diagnosed. In the future, research geared toward identifying if and how mental stress risk assessment may influence mortality from heart disease, what types of interventions are most effective for individuals showing specific symptoms, and whether treating psychosocial factors reduces risk can be expected. Preventative interventions based on cognitive-behavior theories of depression may provide new insight into reducing the associated risks of both depression and heart disease.[54]

# CHAPTER 9

# Women and Heart Disease

In Joy's family, several individuals had suffered heart attacks in their fifties and early sixties despite eating a healthy diet. Joy's mother was in her mid-sixties when she died of a heart attack. A number of her relatives had diabetes. When Joy came to the United States from her family's homeland in Asia, she informed her new doctor of her family medical history. Joy received no information about precautions she could take to lessen her own risk of a heart attack. Her doctor did not tell her about the importance of diet or exercise in preventing heart disease, nor did the doctor mention anything else Joy could do to protect her heart.

Joy was skinny and assumed this meant she would not have a heart attack. To be safe, she had a cholesterol test and found that her overall cholesterol was borderline high. On reaching menopause, her doctor put her on estrogen as a precaution against heart disease and osteoporosis. She thought she had done everything right to avoid a heart attack—she was thin, did not have diabetes, and was taking hormone replacement therapy. And as a woman, she knew her risks were lower than for a man.

After being involved in an automobile accident, Joy felt chronically fatigued, and then her hair began to thin, her skin became dryer, and she lost her eyebrows. She assumed this was all a sign of aging, but her doctor said she had a thyroid disease. As a result of the disease, her cholesterol had risen, and her HDL cholesterol (good cholesterol) had fallen. Soon after receiving medication to stabilize her thyroid condition, she found out she also had another disease that caused spasms in the small arteries in her hands and feet. In rare cases, she was told, this disease could also cause spasms of the coronary artery, leading to a heart attack. Her physician treated her with medicine, including a statin drug.

One day, Joy experienced chest pain while exercising and went to the doctor, who referred her to a cardiologist. Joy's electrocardiogram showed that her heart might not be getting enough blood, so she underwent an additional echocardiogram test. Because the results of this test were negative, her cardiologist told her this meant she did not have coronary artery disease. Six months later, she had a heart attack. Her emergency coronary angiogram showed that three of her coronary arteries were severely blocked.

She underwent successful bypass surgery but had some complications that affected her airway and voice. When she left the hospital, she received little in the way of helpful information about cardiac rehabilitation. She eventually enrolled in a rehabilitation program, at the urging of a friend. The rehabilitation program, run by experienced and knowledgeable nurses, has since played an important role in her life and helped her recover.[1]

Joy's experience is all too common for women. Lack of information on preventing heart disease, missed signs and the complicating presence of other diseases with old age, inaccurate tests, unique complications after bypass surgery, and the failure of medical care practitioners to suggest enrollment in a cardiac rehabilitation program are just a few of the problems that many women face when dealing with heart disease.

Because heart disease mortality for men has traditionally been substantially higher than for women, perceptions of the public and even the medical profession have tended to discount the real risks that women face. Yet, in the last decade, the government, public health agencies, and medical organizations have made major efforts to rectify the past inattention to women. This chapter reviews some of the misunderstandings about women's heart disease, the difference in the nature and treatment of heart disease among women and men, and the progress made in recent decades to deal with women's special problems.

## THE MALE MODEL OF HEART DISEASE

Heart disease remains the number-one killer of both men and women in the United States. Surprisingly to most people, it poses a much greater danger than any other disease, including cancer, to the health of Americans. At birth, the probability of eventually dying from major coronary vascular disease is 47 percent, compared with 22 percent for cancer.[2] Despite the prevalence of heart disease in the population overall, most Americans have a dangerously naive understanding of the disease. Outdated generalizations on who is at risk from heart disease, what its symptoms are, and how it is treated dominate the public's attitude about this killer.

The most familiar image of a person suffering heart disease is a man experiencing a crushing, burning pain in his chest that may spread to his arms or throat. Physical exertion—moving heavy objects, for example— often triggers the discomfort. As a result, the man is likely to end up at a hospital, with a doctor explaining the results of a noninvasive test, such as an electrocardiogram test, that measures how well the heart is functioning. Preparing for the future, the man is told about lifestyle changes he must make to rehabilitate his heart, and he may be prescribed medication. This "male model" of heart disease is what most people, regardless of their sex, envision as typical—unfortunately, it is not accurate for all people, and it may understate the real danger that heart disease presents to those with atypical symptoms.

The male model of heart disease fits the experience of many patients with heart disease and the observations of doctors about most of their patients. Yet the model is not universal. Some men who suffer from heart disease experience different symptoms or no symptoms at all before a heart event. In fact, 50 percent of men who die suddenly of coronary heart disease have no previous symptoms.[3] Worse, the male model does not fit women. While a woman may feel chest pain similar to that experienced by many men, women more often feel discomfort in the abdomen, shoulder, arm, neck, or back and experience shortness of breath. These symptoms, typically associated with problems other than heart disease, are often dismissed as related to a stomach ache, mild sickness, or age-related discomforts. Moreover, 63 percent of women who die suddenly of coronary heart disease had no previous symptoms.[4]

The implications of the male model are that many people, and especially women, misunderstand, fail to recognize, and often do not treat either the threat or the symptoms of heart disease. A 1997 survey of more than a thousand women found that as few as 8 percent believed heart disease and stroke are the greatest health threat to women. About 90 percent did not know that nausea, fatigue, and dizziness are warning signals of a heart attack in women. Approximately half of the women surveyed knew that postmenopausal women are more likely than men to have heart attacks. Less than one-third reported that their doctor talked about heart disease when discussing general health, and only 18 percent recalled seeing, hearing, or reading anything about heart disease in their health care professional's office in the last year.[5] These dismal findings are only the tip of the iceberg when it comes to misconceptions about women and heart disease.

## BASIC FACTS ABOUT WOMEN AND HEART DISEASE

Heart disease in the United States kills more women than the next seven leading causes of death combined, and one woman dies from heart disease each minute. Approximately 1 in 2.4 women's deaths result from heart disease, while 1 in 29 deaths result from breast cancer.[6] Experts calculate that one in five females have some form of cardiovascular disease. Cardiovascular diseases killed 505,661 females in the United States in 2000, compared with 267,009 females who died of all forms of cancer combined and compared with 440,175 males who died of cardiovascular disease.[7]

Women and older people have often been underrepresented in studies that examine heart disease and its risk factors. The exclusion of women from many of these studies has compromised their quality of care and health safety.[8] In the mid-1990s, a major study showed that during routine visits to doctors' offices, women received less counseling about exercise, nutrition, and weight reduction—all crucial components of managing heart disease risk—than men did. Furthermore, doctors have tended to miss opportunities to reduce heart disease and control risk factors in female patients that they are not likely to miss in male patients. After a myocardial infarction or bypass surgery, for example, doctors often recommend that male patients enroll in a heart rehabilitation program for risk-factor management. Studies have shown women are less likely than men to get a referral to, enroll in, and complete these programs.[9]

Men's hearts and women's hearts work in basically the same way and do not differ anatomically from each other. Yet women live an average of seven years longer than men, and heart disease generally appears a decade later in women than in men. Women's longer life expectancy compared with men's may be associated with later onset of heart disease, but it also complicates the diagnosis and treatment of heart disease. Heart disease in women often manifests in ways unlike that described by the male model. Older age leaves the body more fragile and less able to heal itself. Osteoporosis, arthritis, or other chronic ailments are often present in addition to heart disease, and other diseases that foster heart disease, such as hypertension and diabetes, are also more likely present. Additionally, women tend to experience symptoms at rest or during emotional strain instead of during or immediately following physical activity. These factors and others can complicate diagnosis and treatment of heart disease in women.

Primary risk factors such as smoking, family history, lack of physical activity, overweight and obesity, high cholesterol, and diabetes apply to both men and women. Other factors—ethnicity, sex, and gender, among others—can play a role in mitigating or magnifying the effects of the primary risk factors.

Female biology and the way it changes over the life cycle play a specific role in heart risk that is unique to women. Estrogen and other factors afford women in the reproductive stages of their lives a natural protection against the brunt of heart disease's effects. Yet as women age, their risk of heart disease rises significantly.[10] Before menopause, estrogen helps

maintain normal blood vessel response to stress in women. After menopause, a woman's risk increases due to the effect of falling levels of estrogen on blood vessel function and blood-clotting factors.

Some investigators have suggested that women's changing social roles
over the last several decades explain why women's death rates from heart
disease have not fallen as quickly as men's have. The gender-specific pressures young women may feel—to be thin, for example—can promote un-
healthful dietary habits, a tendency to smoke, and less leisure-time
physical activity. Studies have shown that males and females begin smoking and continue smoking for different reasons, and weight gain associated with quitting smoking may affect the choice to stop. Since heart
disease is a disease that develops over a lifetime, early behavior patterns
can have a large influence on later progression of heart disease. Women
with heart disease may also experience greater levels of social isolation
because of being older, outliving their spouses, and living alone. Elderly
and minority women often have less access to health care and are less
likely to receive preventative care, in many cases because they cannot
afford regular visits to the doctor or they are not covered by private health
insurance to supplement public Medicare services. Women's health complaints also tend to be taken less seriously than men's complaints during
doctor visits.[11]

The differences in treating heart disease in women compared with men
often result from missed or misinterpreted signs and symptoms. Starting
with the initial diagnosis, clinicians and patients often attribute chest
pains in women to noncardiac causes. While both women and men may
show typical chest pain that grips the chest and spreads to the shoulders,
neck, or arms, women may have a greater tendency than men to have
atypical chest pain or to complain of abdominal pain, difficulty breathing,
nausea, and unexplained fatigue. Not expecting, not knowing, or denying
the possibility that their symptoms are those typical of heart attacks,
women may also avoid or delay seeking medical care. Another confound-
ing factor for both women and physicians may be that, since women tend
to have heart attacks later in life than men do, other conditions that can
mask heart attack symptoms are often present. Once heart disease is diagnosed, both age and the more advanced stage of coronary disease in
women can affect the availability of treatment options. These factors may
also explain the greater mortality of women after heart attacks.[12]

Not all the diagnostic tests and procedures designed for and made
available to men are as accurate in women, and physicians may not use
them for that reason. As a result, physicians may detect the coronary process in women leading up to a heart attack or stroke too late, and later
intervention and more serious consequences result. The exercise stress
test, for example, may be less accurate in women. This test can give a false
positive result in young women with a low likelihood of coronary heart

disease, and it may not pick up single-vessel heart disease, which is more common in women than in men. More precise and less invasive diagnostic tests such as stress nuclear imaging scans and stress echocardiography are more expensive. Newer technologies such as electron-beam computed tomography (or ultrafast CT) do not yet have well-defined predictive value and cost-effectiveness.[13]

The times near pregnancy and the 10-year period around menopause present unique opportunities for preventative intervention and risk reduction in women. These periods in a woman's life provide an ideal and unique time for obstetricians, gynecologists, and other physicians to review a woman's risk for heart disease, including her overall health and behavior pattern. Because women are likely to see their doctors regularly at these times, medical professionals should use these visits to review women's overall lifestyle for risk factors and to inform women about the real risk that heart disease poses to them.

For postmenopausal women, doctors are exploring estrogen replacement therapy as an option for combating heart disease. This therapy, however, has many possible risks.[14] Two major studies on this topic found contradictory results, and one of them terminated early because of an observed link between hormone replacement therapy and increased risk of heart attack, breast cancer, blood clots, and strokes. The Nurses' Health Study, one of the major long-term observational studies on women's health, had earlier found that women using hormones had 30 percent fewer heart attacks. In contrast, the recent Women's Health Initiative examined randomly selected women and was ended when one of the most widely used hormone replacement drugs, Prempro, had risks that outweighed its benefits—women taking the drug had 40 percent more heart attacks than those taking a placebo. Both studies are supported by the finding that women with heart disease had further increased risk after taking estrogen.[15]

## NEW RESEARCH EFFORTS

Most of the major cardiovascular research studies were conducted on men and neglected women. Women of child-bearing age are at low risk for heart disease, and older women often suffer from other chronic ailments that made the separate study of heart disease difficult. However, clinical studies are now underway to bridge the gap between men and women. They should begin to clarify the sex and gender differences that affect the sources, diagnosis, and treatment of women and men with heart disease.

The National Institutes of Health (NIH), the primary source of funding for medical research, has responded in important ways to the understudy of women. In 1990, the NIH instituted a policy of including women and minority groups in all human-subject research. In 1993, revised guidelines strengthened the 1990 policy statement by affirming that women and minority groups were to be included in all biomedical and behavioral studies. They also mandated that clinical trials must include women and minorities in ways that allow valid analyses of differences in intervention effect across groups, that cost is not a valid reason for excluding these groups, and that effort must be made to initiate programs and outreach to recruit these groups for studies. "It is the policy of NIH that women and members of minority groups and their subpopulations must be included in all NIH-funded clinical research, unless a clear and compelling rationale and justification establishes . . . that inclusion is inappropriate with respect to the health of the subjects or the purpose of the research." Since the early 1990s, NIH-funded research on heart disease has included women, and it will continue to do so in the future, assuring that issues regarding women and minorities' health will not be overlooked as they were in the early studies.[16]

## A FEMINIST VIEW

The attention traditionally given to males in medical research on heart disease ostensibly results from the higher rates of premature mortality among males. However, many feminists argue that the neglect of research on women represents something more troubling, that it stems from the lack of power of women in medical schools and the medical profession. The Feminist Majority Foundation, in calling for equality between men and women in the social and political realms, gives much attention in their agenda to the goal of medical equality.[17] As women's lives depend on their treatment in clinics and hospitals, eliminating inequality in the medical system is an integral part of larger efforts to promote feminism.

The Feminists Majority Foundation notes that despite a rising number of female medical students (now about 36 percent of all students), women make up only a small part of the leadership of medical schools and the medical profession. According to the foundation, the resulting lack of power of women—and the presence of the special perspective they bring—accounts for the neglect of women in research. "Feminist women in medicine make a profound difference in not only what medical technologies are used, but also in the way doctors view their patients as human beings. . . . Women, by their very presence, bring a perspective and a value system to their environment far different from the male-dominated view that has persisted for so long."[18]

Much room remains for improvement in medical equality for men and women. The Feminist Majority Foundation calls for integration of women's perspectives into medical school curricula, gender balance at all levels of the school, and comprehensive testing of the effectiveness of new products on women as well as men.[19]

## SEVEN MYTHS ABOUT HEART DISEASE

Despite greater knowledge of the differences in heart disease between men and women, and efforts to include women in more medical studies, myths about heart disease in women persist. Foremost among the common myths is that heart disease is a man's disease.[20] Estrogen does offer women a degree of protection from heart disease during their reproductive years, but after age 60, one in four women will die of heart disease—the same ratio at which men die. Furthermore, estrogen may not offer the same protection to women with diabetes and with genetic risk for premature heart disease.

A second myth holds that cancer is more of a threat to women than heart disease. Actually, twice as many women die each year of cardiovascular disease as die of all forms of cancer combined, and six times more women die of coronary artery disease, the single most lethal type of heart disease for women, than die of breast cancer.

The third widely believed myth is that only older women have to worry about heart disease. One in seven women between ages 45 and 64 have had heart disease or a stroke. The behaviors that contribute to the development of heart disease in both women and men are linked to patterns that often begin relatively early in life. Many adult smokers began in their teens; overeating, eating non-nutritious foods, and failing to exercise regularly are also habits that often start in youth and carry over into adulthood.

A fourth myth is that chest pain is a normal part of aging. Chest pain indicates a health problem. Along with anxiety, depression, gallbladder problems, bronchitis, and indigestion, heart disease is one of many health problems resulting in chest pain. Women more than men tend to assume their chest pain is caused by something other than heart disease, but missing this symptom can lead to late diagnosis, progression of the disease, and death.

A fifth myth has many people believing that a basic cholesterol test is adequate for determining women's risk of developing heart disease. As many as 80 percent of people who have heart attacks also have cholesterol levels within the normal range, and three other risk factors emerge particularly important for postmenopausal women—high LDL cholesterol, low HDL cholesterol, and high triglyceride levels. A lipid profile of all three of these factors supplies a more accurate indication of a woman's risk than the level of total cholesterol alone. Even a full lipid profile fails to take account of other risk factors such as smoking or a sedentary lifestyle.

A sixth myth—that heart disease patients receive the same treatment whether male or female—can lead to assumptions about care that may have drastic consequences on women's health. For women more than men, heart disease tends to be diagnosed later in life, to be more serious when diagnosed, and to be treated less aggressively.

The seventh commonly believed myth is that men and women benefit equally from the same types of treatment. Women require different methods of screening for heart disease. Women die more often than men during bypass surgery and tend to fare worse from other, less-invasive procedures as well. Women do not get as much relief from their symptoms as men when undergoing the same treatments, and women suffer more complications than men after some of the same procedures.

Together, these seven myths account for a great deal of the misunderstanding that has prevented women from benefiting as much as men from the last 50 years of progress against heart disease.

## WHAT MAKES WOMEN'S HEART DISEASE DIFFERENT

Since the 1950s, the progress observed in declining death rates from heart disease has been slower for women than for men.[21] Smoking rates are declining less for women than for men, the prevalence of obesity is rising among women (and men), and a large majority of women participate in little or no leisure-time physical activity. More than half of women over age 45 have elevated blood pressure, and approximately 40 percent of women over age 55 have high cholesterol.[22] These conditions are prime areas for intervention and offer hope that the dangers of heart disease for women can be further diminished by some relatively easy-to-take steps.

Throughout their lifetimes, women tend to have higher levels of HDL cholesterol than men, and from their teens into their fifties, women also tend to have lower LDL cholesterol. These are positive factors working in women's favor that scientists believe are linked to natural estrogen. Estrogen in women helps keep LDL cholesterol low and favorably influences the heart and circulatory system. Testosterone in men raises LDL cholesterol and lowers HDL cholesterol, perhaps accounting for earlier heart disease in men than women.

Hormone activity also determines the progression of heart disease in women. After menopause, estrogen levels fall and women's LDL cholesterol climbs an average of 25 points—a significant amount. Early menopause before age 35 confers two to three times the risk of having a heart attack compared with women the same age who have a later menopause. Removal of ovaries before age 35 raises the risk of heart attack by a factor of seven because ovaries produce estrogen.[23] The effects of female hormones, especially estrogen, on the development of heart disease highlights the need for different strategies to treat heart disease in women.

Many women worry about taking birth-control pills that contain estrogen, having heard of the increased risk of heart disease and stroke. Once thought that birth-control pills increased heart risk, further research revealed that the increased heart risk earlier attributed to the pill was actually linked to smoking. Today's birth-control pills contain far less estrogen than the earlier versions. No studies associate long-term risk for heart disease and use of birth-control pills, although hypertension is more prevalent in women taking the pill.

Other factors considered relevant for female heart risk are pregnancy and body size. For a short time, pregnancy adds stress on the heart and blood vessels by raising blood lipids, insulin, and blood-sugar levels. Usually, these factors do not persist long enough to cause permanent deterioration of a woman's health. However, women who have been pregnant six or more times have a significantly increased heart risk compared with other women.[24] Since the female body is generally smaller than the male body, female hearts and arteries also are smaller. Thus, less plaque may create blockages in the blood vessels, and male time lines do not apply identically to women.

Minority women have a particularly high risk for heart disease.[25] The death rate of black women with cardiovascular disease is 69 percent greater than for white women with the disease. Black women also tend to have more coronary artery disease than black men, while the opposite is true among whites. During the 1980s and 1990s, deaths from heart disease among white women dropped more rapidly than deaths in black women. The higher prevalence of diabetes and obesity among black women compared with white women is thought to explain some of this disparity. Mexican Americans have higher rates of hospitalization for heart attacks compared to non-Hispanic whites, for both men and women. Rates of death after heart attacks are also higher in Mexican Americans compared with non-Hispanic whites, as they are for women compared with men.[26]

---

### SEX AND GENDER IN HEART DISEASE

In discussing differences between men and women, scholars often distinguish between factors relating to sex and gender. Sex is used to refer to biological differences between men and women, while gender is used to refer to learned psychological, social, cultural, and lifestyle differences between men and women. Both have important roles in accounting for patterns of heart disease, but gender-based lifestyle factors more than biological factors can be changed to improve the health of both men and women.

To illustrate, consider differences across nations. In the United States, 53 women die of coronary heart disease per 100 men; in Sweden, 44 women died per 100 men; and in France, 38 women die per 100 men.[27] Relative to males, then, females have greater protection from heart disease in France than in Sweden, and in Sweden than in the United States. Can biological

differences in women account for this variation? It seems unlikely that estrogen levels vary greatly across the countries. The essential biology of
women does not change drastically across national borders. However, the
social behavior and lifestyles of men and women can vary greatly across the
nations. For example, cigarette use of women relative to men is lower in
France than the other nations and might account for low female heart disease
there. Other gender-based factors relating to diet and stress might also be
important. Sex-based or biological factors certainly contribute to the lower
rates of heart disease among women, but the variations across nations suggest that environment factors are crucial as well. Identification of these factors can play an important role in public health policies that aims to reduce
female heart disease.

## MEASURING THE EFFECTS OF HEART DISEASE
## ON WOMEN

Each year since 1984, more females than males have died of heart disease in the United States. While the number of male deaths has declined
from more than 500,000 in 1980 to approximately 444,000 in 2000, the
number of female deaths has increased from approximately 470,000 in
1979 to more than 500,000 in 2000. Although overall rates of death from
heart disease for both men and women have declined over this same period, in 2000, 53.5 percent of total deaths from heart disease were females.
Men and women between ages 65 and 74 experience approximately the
same prevalence of cardiovascular disease—before those ages, men have
higher prevalence. After age 74, prevalence is higher in women.[28] The
lifetime risk of developing heart disease after age 40 is 49 percent for men
and 32 percent for women, at age 70 it is only 35 percent for men and 24
percent for women.[29] Although the change over the life course may reflect
the earlier death of men from heart disease, it also emphasizes the point
that heart illnesses and risk factors affect women in particular ways.

### Coronary Heart Disease

Coronary heart disease killed 254,630 American women in 2000, representing 49 percent of all such deaths. From 1970 to 2000, hospital discharges of females with diagnosed coronary heart disease increased 49
percent. Death is but one outcome that must be accounted for in measuring the effects of heart disease on women. About 6.6 million females alive
in 2003 had a heart attack, angina, or both. A heart attack or stroke causes
most sudden deaths in America and heart attacks or strokes also cause
higher mortality than other illnesses. Female heart attack victims face
worse odds than male victims. Women are more likely than men to die

from a heart attack within a few weeks after the event, in large part because they tend to have heart attacks at an older age. Of the estimated 210,000 women who will have a heart attack this year, including both first-time and recurrent events, 38 percent will die within a year. Approximately 25 percent of men who have a heart attack die within one year.[30] Almost half of men and women under age 65 who have a heart attack die within eight years. Within six years after a recognized heart attack, 18 percent of men and 35 percent of women will have another heart attack, 7 percent of men and 6 percent of women will die suddenly from causes related to heart disease, and 22 percent of men and 46 percent of women will be disabled with heart failure.[31]

The average age at which women have their first heart attack is 70.4; for men, it is age 65.8. In 2000, approximately 44,000 Americans between ages 29 and 44 had heart attacks, with men having 3.4 times more than women. Among those aged 45 to 64, 343,000 had heart attacks, with men having almost 3.0 times more than women. Among those aged 65 and older, 744,000 had heart attacks, with men having 1.4 times more than women.[32] Heart attacks often lead to potentially deadly strokes—approximately 8 percent of men and 11 percent of women will have a stroke within six years of a heart attack.[33]

### Heart Failure

Two-and-a-half million American women have congestive heart failure today.[34] Before age 75, most heart events in women are due to congestive heart failure.[35] Risks of heart failure for women differ from men. Diabetes is a stronger risk factor for women, especially younger women, than for men, and obesity has a greater predictive value of heart failure for women, but total cholesterol is significant only for men. Smoking is a less-common factor in heart failure in female than in male patients, but hypertension appears to increase women's risk more than men's risk. After a heart attack, women are more likely than men to develop heart failure.[36] Approximately 22 percent of males and 46 percent of females became disabled by heart failure within six years of a heart attack.[37]

Women with heart failure have a poorer quality of life than men because women have lower baseline physical health and show less improvement in the first year after onset of heart failure. They also appear to show more symptoms and signs of heart failure, including swelling (edema) and poorer exercise tolerance. In the United Kingdom, Sweden, New Zealand, the United States, and the Netherlands, surveys have shown that at younger ages, men are admitted and discharged from hospitals from heart failure at a higher rate than women with the difference diminishing as age increases. But because older women represent a large portion of the population, more women are hospitalized for heart failure with longer hospital stays.[38] Despite their longer hospital stays and greater number of hospitalizations, however, female patients with congestive heart failure appear to have a better prognosis than male patients do.[39]

### Diabetes

Of 16.6 million Americans estimated to have diagnosed or undiagnosed diabetes, 8.6 million are women. About 5.9 million of these women have been diagnosed by their physician and another 2.7 million are undiagnosed. In addition, about 5.6 million females are among the estimated 14.2 million Americans with prediabetes.[40] Out of 210,000 deaths from diabetes in 2000, 54.4 percent were females, with 75 percent of all diabetic deaths related to heart or blood vessel diseases.[41] Diabetes increases risk of coronary heart disease in women by three to seven times compared with two to three times in men.[42] In middle-aged men, diabetes increases cardiovascular disease death risk five times. For middle-aged women with diabetes, the risk is eight times greater than for women without the disease.[43] In part, this may be because diabetes diminishes the protective benefits of estrogen.[44] Yet, one recent study questioned whether diabetes actually causes increased risk of heart disease in the women and suggested that other factors such as smoking, overweight, and obesity may account for the higher risk of heart disease among diabetic women.[45]

### High Blood Pressure

About one in five Americans has high blood pressure, and 25 percent of American adults do.[46] In 2000, 26,685 females died from high blood pressure, representing 59.8 percent of total deaths from high blood pressure. A higher percentage of men than women have high blood pressure until age 55. Between ages 55 and 74, the percentage of women is slightly higher than of men, and after that, the percentage is much higher. Some women are at particularly high risk from high blood pressure. Women who take birth control pills are two to three times more likely to have high blood pressure than women who do not. Black women make ambulatory hospital visits for hypertension 85 percent more often than white women.

### Risk Factors

Greater risks of heart disease appear in older women who have high cholesterol levels. A higher percentage of women aged 50 and older have a total blood cholesterol of 200 mg/dL or higher than men of the same age (200 mg/dL to 239 mg/dL is considered borderline high risk; 240

mg/dL and above is high risk). In 2000, 55 million adult women had total blood cholesterol levels that were high risk or borderline high risk. Triglyceride levels also may be particularly significant indicators of risk in women.[47]

Women, the elderly, non-Hispanic blacks, and Hispanics participate in less physical activity than other groups, thus increasing their risk of heart disease. Married women are more likely than other women to engage in at least some leisure-time physical activity. Psychosocial stress is more likely than physical exertion to trigger sudden cardiac arrest in women, while for men the opposite is true.[48] The Nurses Health Study found that women who maintain healthy lifestyles, including regular exercise, not smoking, a normal weight, better diet, and moderate consumption of alcohol, lower their risk of coronary heart disease compared with women who do not.[49] Among women with heart disease, marital stress—but not work stress—appears to impact prognosis negatively in women ages 30 to 65 years. A study in Stockholm, Sweden, found that among women married or cohabiting with a male partner, marital stress increased the risk for recurrent heart events.[50] More study of all these factors is needed to design programs of prevention, diagnosis, and treatment specifically for women.

## POTENTIAL FOR IMPROVEMENT

Knowledge is the best tool when it comes to combating disease effectively, and until recently, most knowledge gained about heart disease has been gathered from male test subjects. However, strides to correct this imbalance include requiring both male and female subjects in federally funded research. Large long-term studies of women that contribute to our understanding of the causes and outcomes of heart disease should prove useful to reduce the rate of female heart disease mortality.

With a new knowledge base, public health experts hope to encourage women to take a more active role in monitoring their heart risk. Women are advised to routinely have mammograms in order to help catch breast disease. A similar impetus to monitor heart risks can help women benefit fully from medical advances. Because physicians rely on their patients to communicate information on their current health status, increased knowledge among women about heart disease can help them communicate more effectively with their doctors. The more women know about the special symptoms they experience from heart disease such as nausea and fatigue, the better they can communicate this information.

Women with heart disease can also do more to help in their own treatment. Studies have shown that following many types of heart events women have a worse prognosis than men, especially after a heart attack or bypass surgery. Despite the effectiveness of rehabilitation programs, women do not take advantage of them to the degree that men do. They attend programs less often and drop out more often than men.[51] The action of women to learn more about heart problems and participate in rehabilitation can help reduce female deaths from heart disease at a faster rate.

# PART IV

## Past and Future

# CHAPTER 10

# Twentieth-Century Trends

In 1948, Americans could celebrate the three-year anniversary of victory in World War II over Germany and Japan with a sense that long periods of peace and prosperity would follow. The economy had started a postwar growth that would lead to ever-higher standards of living for most Americans. Optimism and confidence in the future would soon lead to the high birth rates of the baby boom. President Truman ended racial segregation in the military, and Jackie Robinson began his second year with the Brooklyn Dodgers as the first African American Major League Baseball player. The American military, although threatened by communism in Eastern Europe and Southeast Asia, was recognized as the world's strongest.

That same year may be seen as a turning point in the fight against heart disease. After rising for the first half of the century, heart disease in 1948 continued as the major killer of Americans. Despite continued progress in dealing with infectious diseases, rising mortality rates from heart disease did not slow. Reflecting their considerable anxiety about the situation, public health officials called the steady increase an epidemic of coronary heart disease. To address the epidemic, the United States Congress passed a bill to establish the National Heart Institute. The bill referred to the "gross underemphasis on cardiovascular research" and noted that "only about 7 cents per death is now being spent on research in cardiovascular disease."[1] With an initial allocation of $500,000, the National Heart Institute began to conduct and coordinate research on cardiovascular disease.

When President Truman signed the bill into law in June 1948, the prospects for dealing with the problems of heart disease appeared dim. At that time, a heart attack meant certain death for about a third of all victims.

Survivors faced six weeks in a hospital, treatment with little more than painkillers and rest, and six more months in bed at home; many had to go on disability retirement after a heart attack.[2]

It took more than another decade after the founding of the National Heart Institute for deaths from heart disease to begin dropping, but the national efforts signified by the founding led to the progress that we have enjoyed in recent decades. In the half century since 1948, the institute promoted research on treatment and diagnostic methods that have become commonplace. The institute also funded studies to identify the major risk factors for heart disease and educate the public about those risks. In so doing, it would contribute to an extraordinary decline in heart disease mortality over the last part of the twentieth century.

Today, the renamed National Heart, Lung, and Blood Institute receives nearly 2 billion dollars a year for research and education, and can take credit for much of the progress we have made against heart disease. As the current director of the institute states, "We have much to celebrate. The nation's investment in heart science has paid off in ways that could not have been imagined."[3]

This chapter provides an overview of the progress made against heart disease by describing the trends in heart disease mortality both before and after the time of the founding of the National Heart Institute. It reviews how heart disease rose in the early part of the twentieth century and then fell in the late part as medical treatments and social lifestyles improved. It also notes the instances where progress has been less than desired and identifies areas of needed improvement.

## THE RISE AND FALL OF HEART DISEASE

Most of human history has been characterized by plague and famine. People not only faced early death and high mortality in the best of circumstances, but they also suffered from periodic disease epidemics and food shortages that further shortened their lives. With industrialization, improved standards of living, and better nutrition, infectious diseases as causes of death receded, and devastating epidemics declined. These changes led to the low and stable mortality rates enjoyed in most modern societies. Death now occurs most often at older ages from diseases that involve the wearing down and malfunctioning of the human organism rather than from infectious diseases.[4]

Heart disease has become the major cause of death in the modern era. Uncommon a hundred years ago when death came from contagious epidemics, poor nutrition, and childhood maladies, heart disease emerged as the number-one killer in the United States and most affluent nations. Heart disease reflects a process of wearing out or malfunctioning. Rare among children and young people but frequent at older ages, heart disease involves the steady accumulation of small problems into larger ones as, over the years, arteries to the heart clog and the valves and muscles of the heart weaken.

In the Netherlands, heart disease represented only 4 percent of all deaths in 1880, but at its peak in 1970, it had reached 33 percent.[5] The increase stemmed not just from the greater incidence of heart problems but also from the decline of other sorts of infectious diseases that caused many deaths in the nineteenth century. As people survived longer because of the receding epidemics, they faced increasing risks of heart disease.

In the United States, the same upward trend occurred in the early part of the twentieth century. Although changing definitions hinder comparisons over time, it appears that diseases of the heart began a 30- to 40-year rise in 1920.[6] Deaths due to heart disease rose from 8 percent of all deaths in 1910 to 30 percent of all deaths in 1945.[7] Again, part of the increased proportion comes simply from the fewer deaths caused by infectious diseases. In addition, however, the upward trend in the first part of the century involved a real rise of mortality rates from heart disease, particularly among middle and older age groups.[8]

Since the 1960s, the upward trend has reversed at most ages. The decline occurred more strongly among middle-aged persons than older persons, and as a result, heart disease in the United States has become more concentrated in the older ages.[9] The same pattern occurred in the Netherlands, where mortality from heart disease fell steadily from 1970 to 1992.[10] The mid- to late-century reversal of the rise in heart disease seems typical of advanced industrial nations throughout the world.

Some dispute the validity of statistics that show an epidemic rise in heart disease early in the twentieth century and a fall since then.[11] Instead, physicians may simply have become more aware and familiar with the diagnosis of heart disease and used it more often. Conversely, certain previously common categories of death such as apoplexy, "old age," and ill-defined causes declined as official diagnoses. Those changes could account for the rise in heart disease until the 1960s, and a reverse process could account for the more recent decline in heart disease. In the last several decades, advances in making accurate diagnoses might shift the classification of deaths from the heart disease category to other categories. One proponent of this view thus states that statistics on cause of death are too unreliable to identify trends over the last century.[12]

Although such claims remind us of the ever-present risks of error in determining the causes of death, the evidence indicates that meaningful changes have in fact occurred in mortality from heart disease. If the changes came only from errors of reporting and classifying deaths, they should affect men and women in much the same way. Yet, as the discussion to follow will indicate, male death from heart disease rose at a faster pace from 1920 to 1950 than female deaths. Since changes in determining the cause of death should not differ for men and women, the different changes in death from heart disease for men and women contradict the claim that increases in heart disease during that period resulted solely from errors in identifying causes of death. Even allowing for the bias in death certificates, heart disease (particularly among males) has grown in importance during this period.[13]

Concerning the more recent decline in heart disease mortality, a 1978 conference sponsored by the National Heart, Lung, and Blood Institute determined that the decline since 1968 was real; another conference in 1986 confirmed that finding.[14] If anything, changes in measurement in recent years may have moderated the decline in heart disease. For example, a 1968 revision in the International Classification of Disease led to a 13 percent increase in classified coronary or ischemic heart disease.[15] Yet the downward pattern continued after this change. More recent changes in the International Classification of Disease also reclassify some forms of heart disease but again lead to only small changes in the downward trend. The decline in heart disease mortality since the 1960s can be described as large, real, and consistent.[16]

## THE NATIONAL INSTITUTES OF HEALTH

The National Institutes of Health (NIH), the major source of government funding for research on health and the umbrella organization for the National Heart, Lung, and Blood Institute, traces its roots back to 1887. In that year, Joseph J. Kinyoun founded the Hygienic Laboratory, an off-shoot of the Marine Hospital, and it eventually became the Public Health Service. In 1901, the Hygienic Laboratory was recognized when Congress passed a law appropriating $35,000 to pay for a new home for the laboratory to investigate "infectious and contagious diseases and matters pertaining to public health."[17]

During World War I, the Hygienic Laboratory investigated anthrax outbreaks among troops and found that contaminated shaving brushes were to blame. In 1916, the laboratory hired its first woman bacteriologist, Dr. Ida Bengtson. The laboratory was renamed the National Institute of Health in 1930 and given authorization to establish fellowships for the study of basic biological and medical problems. This marked the beginning in the American scientific community of a concerted effort to fund medical research publicly. The National Cancer Institute was formed seven years later and it became a part of the NIH. In 1948 the National Heart Institute was formed, and it has since played a critical role in heart disease research through the projects it has funded. The budget of the NIH expanded from $8 million in 1947 to more than $1 billion in 1966. In 2003, the budget was approximately $27.2 billion, with $2.8 billion of that earmarked for the National Heart, Lung, and Blood Institute for research.

## A LOOK AT THE DOWNWARD TRENDS

To provide some more precise figures on recent changes, 359,423 men and 379,744 women died of heart disease in 1998.[18] Because women make up a larger part of the population than men, the comparison of the numbers of deaths can be misleading. When divided by the male or female population, 272.0 per 100,000 men died of heart disease in 1998, while 274.5 per 100,000 women died. How have these rates changed over time? The mortality rate for males peaked in 1968 at a level of 441.3, while for females it peaked in the same year at 315.9. The trend for males represents a substantial decline of 38.3 percent. The 13.1 percent decline for females has been smaller but still significant. The greater decline among males has equalized sex differences in the mortality rates.

It may appear surprising that the 1998 rates for men and women (272.0 versus 274.5) are nearly identical. However, the faster decline among men and the similar rates in 1998 may result from shifts in the age structure of the population. After the baby boom of the 1950s, the size of the child, youth, and middle-age population grew, making the proportion of persons age 65 and over—those facing the highest risks of heart disease—smaller. Even if the risks of heart disease at particular ages remained constant, changes in the relative sizes of the age groups would reduce the rate of heart disease mortality. More recently, however, the growth of large numbers of baby boomers into late middle age has the potential to do the opposite—inflate the death rate from heart disease. Such influences can, in particular, bias comparisons between men and women. Since women live to older ages, a higher proportion of their population is old and most subject to heart disease. The high proportion of elderly women would raise their rate of heart disease relative to men.

To adjust for shifts in age structure and isolate the influence of changes in the risks of heart disease for those about the same age, one can look at rates within specific age groups. Describing trends among men and women ages 55 to 64 would have two benefits. First, it would compare men and women in the same age groups. Second, it would also focus on ages of premature heart disease mortality rather than on older ages when deaths from all causes become more common.

For males at ages 55–64, a strong downward trend appears. The peak rate of heart disease mortality of 1,089.7 occurred earlier than for all ages—in 1957. By 1998, it had fallen to 411.1 for a 62.3 percent decrease. For females in this age group, the peak occurred in 1957 at 450.5 and has fallen to 173.9 for a 61.4 percent decrease. These changes reflect major reductions in the risks of death for middle aged men and women. Yet, females maintain a substantial advantage in heart disease over males at these ages. Men had rates 2.36 times higher than women in 1998.

Comparisons at other ages show much the same change. At ages 45–

54, heart disease mortality rates fell by 47.8 percent for males and by 37.7 percent for females. At ages 65 to 74, the rates fell by 36.5 for males and by 35.3 percent for females. The declines are generally larger for those in the middle age than for those at the younger and older ages but represent important progress in all three age groups. Females maintain an advantage over males at all ages except for those under age 35. Males have rates over twice as high as females at ages under 65, somewhat higher rates at ages 65–84, and similar rates at ages 85 and over.

In addition to the age-group comparisons, one can also examine age-adjusted rates. The age-adjusted rates are based on calculations that assume the size of age groups in the population does not change or differ by sex, and that only the risks of disease at specific ages change.

In age-adjusted terms, the male rate of heart disease mortality fell from a peak in 1963 of 605.9 to a low point in 1998 of 287.7. This represents a decline of 52.5 percent. For females, the peak of 373.1 in 1957 fell to 175.5 in 1998. The 53.0 percent decline again demonstrates that both men and women have enjoyed improvements. The age-adjusted rates also demonstrate that heart disease mortality among women is lower than for men. The male age-adjusted rate of 287.7 in 1998 exceeds the female age adjusted rate of 175.5 by a factor of 1.64. Women have benefited from the changes much as men have.

### Trends by Type of Heart Disease

Perhaps the trends differ by type of heart disease. Based on the varieties of ways the heart can malfunction, the International Classification of Disease divides deaths from heart disease into several categories.[19] In terms of size, the largest number of deaths comes from coronary heart or artery disease: of all heart disease deaths in 1998, 63 percent come from coronary heart disease.

Along with representing the most important type of heart disease, coronary heart disease has shown the greatest decline in mortality rates over the last 40 years. Between 1979 and 1998, the death rates from coronary or ischemic heart disease for men and women fell by 30.7 percent.

Among the noncoronary types of heart disease, deaths from hypertensive heart disease, rheumatic heart disease, acute and chronic pulmonary disease, and ill-defined or unspecified heart disease have fallen little and make up a larger part of the total now than in the past. Nonetheless, they still represent only a small portion of all deaths from heart disease. Two other forms of heart disease deaths have grown rather than declined. Hospital admissions and deaths from heart failure and atrial fibrillation have climbed steadily.[20] The rise in these conditions may stem from the decline in deaths from other causes, which leaves more people alive to later succumb to the weakening of the heart muscle or arrhythmias.[21] Despite their rise, these components of heart disease remain a small part of the total and do not counter the decline in coronary artery disease.

### A Slowdown in the Decline in Coronary Heart Disease?

In 1999, a government workshop on coronary heart disease found that the decline in heart disease mortality slowed in the 1990s.[22] The report notes the following annual percentage changes in death rates for coronary heart disease in the United States from 1950 to 1997:

| | |
|---|---|
| **1950–1960** | 2.1 |
| **1960–1967** | 0.2 |
| **1970–1978** | − 3.1 |
| **1980–1990** | − 3.3 |
| **1990–1997** | − 2.7 |

The slower rate of decline in the 1990s (− 2.7) than the 1980s (− 3.3) suggests that trends in the future will not be as encouraging as in the past. As the government report states:

Prevalence rates of many risk factors, such as smoking, dietary saturated fat and cholesterol, serum cholesterol, and hypertension, fell until 1990; however, since then, there has been little or no progress, at least in smoking prevalence, physical inactivity, and hypertension control. Moreover, there are several trends suggesting an increase in population risk, including greater dietary intake of calories, a rapid rise in obesity prevalence, and a striking increase in the prevalence of type-2 diabetes. Taken in aggregate, trends in risk factors since 1990 do not seem to be heading toward a reduced risk.[23]

In addition, the lack of health insurance and access to quality heart care for large parts of the population in the United States may contribute to problems of prevention and treatment of heart disease among disadvantaged groups.[24]

However, more recent data indicate that the apparent slowdown in the 1990s has not lasted. Updated figures from the National Heart, Lung, and Blood Institute show that coronary heart disease changed by the following annual average percentages:[25]

| | |
|---|---|
| **1985–1990** | − 3.4 |
| **1990–1995** | − 2.3 |
| **1995–2000** | − 3.3 |

**Figure 10.1**
**Heart Disease Mortality Rates, 1980–1998**

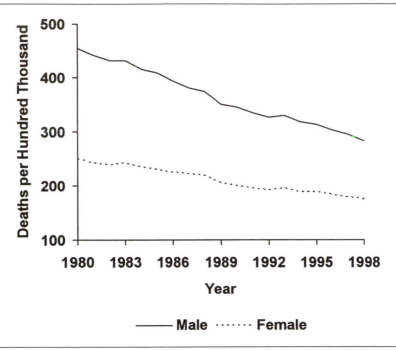

*Source:* World Health Organization, *World Health Statistics Annual* (Geneva, Switzerland: World Health Organization, 1996 and earlier years), http://www.who.int/whosis; Centers for Disease Control and Prevention, *CDC Wonder*, http://wonder.cdc.gov/wonder. (Age-adjusted rates.)

Figure 10.1 further illustrates that there is little evidence of a slowdown. It plots the trends for male and female heart disease mortality (from coronary and other causes) over the time period from 1980 to 1998. The death rates for heart disease in the 1990s declined much as they had in earlier decades.

## MILESTONES IN CARDIOLOGY: 1901–1950

A listing of important events and discoveries in the first part of the twentieth century that have led later to improvements in the treatment of heart disease includes the following.[26]

1901    K. Ingelsrud, a Norwegian surgeon, first uses open-chest cardiac massage to restore a heart to beating.

1903    William Einthoven, a Dutch physiologist, develops the electrocardiograph, a machine to measure the electrical impulses in the heart.

| 1904 | Diastolic blood pressure is first measured by German physiologist Eduard Strasburger. |
| 1905 | The first heart transplant, in a dog, is reported by French-born American biologist, Alexis Carrel. |
| 1908 | S. Saltykow suggests that the presence of high levels of cholesterol in the diet is a cause of atherosclerosis. |
| 1912 | James B. Herrick, an American physician, first describes heart disease resulting from hardening of the arteries. |
| 1913 | Thomas Janeway describes the role of hypertension or high blood pressure in heart failure. |
| 1920 | Harold Pardee, a New York cardiologist, describes the electrocardiographic changes during a heart attack. |
| 1931 | Werner Forssmann of Germany first inserts a catheter into a living heart. |
| 1932 | Solomon A. Hymen of New York describes his use of an artificial pacemaker in animal experiments for heart resuscitation. |
| 1935 | John H. Gibbon, an American cardiovascular surgeon, and his wife build a prototype heart-lung machine. |
| 1937 | Vladimir P. Demikhov, a Soviet scientist, first implants an artificial heart into an animal. |
| 1938 | Robert E. Gross, an American surgeon, performs the first heart surgery. |
| 1942 | H. D. Adams and L. V. Hands of Boston perform the first successful electrical defibrillation of a human. |
| 1948 | Gunnar Jönsson attempts the first coronary angiography. |
| 1950 | Lawrence Craven, a family physician from Cleveland, notes that aspirin can prevent blood clotting. |

## WHO HAS BEEN LEFT BEHIND?

### Race Differences

Although diminishing rates of heart disease mortality have lengthened the lives of men and women, some groups may have benefited more than others. Comparisons across race, for example, disclose that whites have enjoyed the fastest drop in heart disease mortality. The published data on racial differences in mortality go back only to 1979, but the comparisons for even a relatively short time span are revealing. Focusing on age-adjusted rates to avoid the distorting influence of differences among blacks and whites in the proportion of older, high-risk persons in the population, figure 10.2 shows the trends for white males, white females, black males, and black females.

Dropping heart disease mortality, although occurring among all groups, appears largest for white males and then for white females. The advantages of white males relative to black males and of white females relative

**Figure 10.2**
**Race Differences in Heart Disease Mortality Rates, 1979–1998**

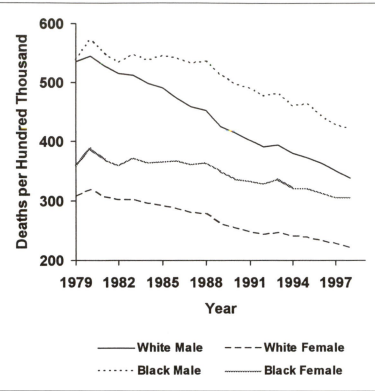

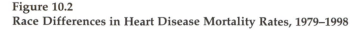

*Source:* World Health Organization, *World Health Statistics Annual* (Geneva, Switzerland: World Health Organization, 1996 and earlier years), http://www.who.int/whosis; Centers for Disease Control and Prevention. *CDC Wonder*, http://wonder.cdc.gov/wonder. (Age-adjusted rates.)

to black females widen considerably over time. By 1998, the steep drop among white males, and the slower drop among black females, leaves only a small gap between the two groups. All groups enjoyed declining heart disease, but the faster decline among whites widened the racial gap.[27]

Some of the racial differences in heart disease mortality may, however, stem from problems in the validity of the estimates of heart disease. One critic notes that a larger proportion of deaths to blacks, particularly in the younger age groups, occur outside the hospital than for whites. For lack of better information, these deaths are often attributed to heart disease.[28] In one study that used autopsies to validate cause of death information on coronary heart disease, 33 percent of blacks were misclassified compared with 18 percent of whites. Such differences contribute to the higher rate of heart disease and the lower rate of decline among blacks.

Despite such error, real racial differences in heart disease almost certainly exist. Even with proper classification, black men have higher rates of death from heart disease because of deprived socioeconomic conditions and poorer medical care. As noted in the next section, heart disease appears highest among low socioeconomic status groups. Race disparities in heart disease thus serve as a measure of social, economic, and medical disadvantage rather than as a reflection of genetic or biological differences.

Although the picture looks discouraging for African Americans, other minority groups enjoy an advantage compared with whites. Native Americans, Asians, and Hispanics have lower coronary heart disease than non-Hispanic whites and blacks.[29] For coronary heart disease in the United States, blacks have the highest age-adjusted rate of 186.8 deaths per hundred thousand, followed by whites at 182.8, Hispanics at 124.2, Native Americans at 112.7, and Asians at 100.1. However, a recent study of coronary heart disease among the native population of Ontario, Canada, finds that hospitalizations for heart disease have doubled. Native and immigrant populations that begin adopting Western lifestyles may experience future increases in heart disease.

### Socioeconomic Status Differences

The decline in heart disease has been greatest among socioeconomic status (SES) groups with high education, high prestige jobs, and high income.[30] As high SES brings advantages in many areas of life, it does much the same in preventing heart disease. In addition, the SES of neighborhoods affects the risks of heart disease. Individuals living in disadvantaged neighborhoods have a higher risk of heart disease than residents of advantaged neighborhoods.[31] By encouraging harmful lifestyles, disadvantaged neighborhoods can raise an individual's risk of heart disease.

Ironically, heart disease was once—and perhaps is still today—viewed as most common among high-status executives under a great deal of stress. Heart bypass surgeries for Michael Eisner of Disney/ABC and Jack Welch of GE provide instances of heart problems of well-known and high-status chief executive officers. Despite this image, high SES groups actually have most changed their lifestyles to improve their risks for heart disease and have benefited most from improved medical care. A study of volunteer participants in an American Cancer Society study finds that a high level of education reduces the risk of coronary heart disease but also that educational differences have been increasing.[32] The rising educational differences mean that heart disease today—like most other diseases—increasingly afflicts low SES groups more than high SES groups.

The increasing disadvantage of low SES groups in heart disease has reinforced a widening gap in mortality from all causes of death between low and high SES groups.[33] Because coronary heart disease contributes significantly to total mortality, it further indicates a widening gap in heart disease mortality between the poor and undereducated relative to the wealthy and well educated. Growing SES differences also explain much of the growing racial differences in heart disease. Concerned with these trends, public health officials and health funding agencies have begun to devote more attention to SES and racial differences in medical and epidemiological research.

### Geographical Differences

Comparisons across regions of the United States establish that coronary heart disease has not fallen as much in the South as elsewhere.[34] The decline in heart disease mortality, for example, began in the northeastern United States in the early 1960s but only started around 1970 in the South.[35] Some cities and towns in the South have actually experienced increases in heart disease. There are particularly high rates of death from heart disease in the Mississippi Delta, in Appalachia and the Ohio River Valley, and in the Piedmont areas of Georgia, South Carolina, and North Carolina.[36] Growing geographical diversity in heart disease has accompanied growing SES and racial diversity.

Another dimension of geographical diversity relates to residence in cities, suburbs, and rural areas. The decline in heart disease occurred earlier in cities than rural areas, and residents of rural areas have experienced a slower decline. "Some areas, such as Mississippi, may actually have experienced increasing CHD [coronary heart disease] mortality rates since the late 1980s. Those areas currently left with high CHD mortality are frequently characterized as rural and poor."[37] Higher income in cities may account for the earlier onset of the decline of heart disease, but it is also the case that crowded and poor neighborhoods of large cities experience high rates of heart disease.[38] Thus, widening geographic inequality has occurred not only between urban and rural areas but also within cities.

---

### MILESTONES IN CARDIOLOGY: 1951–1999

More recent important events in the treatment and prevention of heart disease include the following.[39]

1951    Charles Hufnagel, an American surgeon, develops a plastic valve to repair a leaking aortic valve.

1952    F. John Lewis, an American surgeon, performs the first successful open-heart surgery.

1953    American scientists John Bardeen, Walter H. Brattain, and William B. Shockley produce an implantable pacemaker.

1953    John H. Gibbon, an American cardiovascular surgeon, first uses a pump oxygenator to mechanically pump and purify blood during open-heart surgery.

1954    Inge Edler and Carl H. Hertz first use ultrasound to record the continuous movement of the heart wall.

1961    J. R. Jude, an American cardiologist, leads a team performing the first external cardiac massage to restart a heart.

1963    The American Heart Association publishes a report suggesting that reduction of dietary fat could reduce the incidence of heart disease but states that no "final proof" exists for a causal relationship.

1965    Michael DeBakey and Adrian Kantrowitz, American surgeons, implant mechanical devices to help a diseased heart.

1967    Christian Barnard, a South African surgeon, performs the first whole-heart transplant from one person to another.

1973    A study of Eskimos by J. Dyerberg and H. O. Bang suggests that omega-3 fatty acids found in fish, seal, and whale meat protect against heart disease.

1978    H. Ondetti and colleagues demonstrate that medication can effectively and safely treat hypertension.

1982    William DeVries, an American surgeon, implants a permanent artificial heart, designed by Robert Jarvik, into a patient.

1985    Molecular biologists M. S. Brown and J. L. Goldstein receive the Nobel Prize in Medicine for their work on cholesterol and low-density lipoproteins.

1987    A. R. Gruentzig shows in a study that coronary angioplasty has long-term benefits in reducing the incidence of heart attacks.

1988    P. Saikku of Finland publishes a paper suggesting an association between a newly identified strain of bacteria and chronic heart disease.

1992    Cholesterol-lowering drugs are found to bring benefits not only by lowering cholesterol but also by thinning the blood and preventing blood clots.

1998    Jaume Marrugat of Spain finds that women who suffer heart attacks are more likely to die than their male counterparts.

1998    R. J. Furchgott, L. J. Ignaro, and F. Murad receive the Nobel Prize in Medicine for their discovery of the role of nitric oxide as a signaling mechanism in the cardiovascular system.

1999    Stephen Brown of England describes a new type of laser treatment for blocked arteries.

## HOW DOES THE UNITED STATES COMPARE WITH OTHER COUNTRIES?

The decline in heart disease seen in the United States over the last 20 years has also taken place in the other high-income nations of western

Europe, as well as in Japan, New Zealand, Australia, and Canada.[40] Compared with these nations, coronary heart disease mortality rates in the United States rank as the eleventh-lowest among males and fifteenth-lowest among females (see figures 10.3 and 10.4). The southern European nations of France, Italy, Spain, Portugal, and Greece have the lowest death rates, while the northern European nations of Finland, Sweden, Norway, Germany, Ireland, and the United Kingdom have the highest rates. The rates in the United States fall close to those of the nations of northern

**Figure 10.3**
**Country Differences in Male Heart Disease Mortality Rates, 1994–1996**

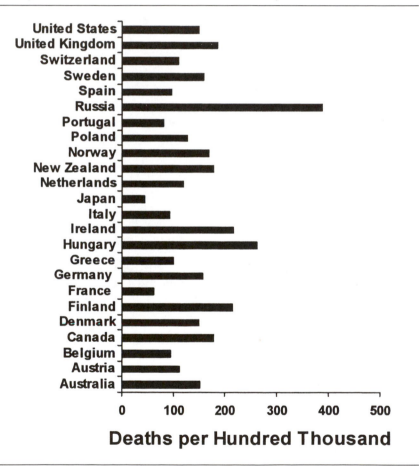

**Deaths per Hundred Thousand**

*Source:* World Health Organization, *World Health Statistics Annual* (Geneva, Switzerland: World Health Organization, 1996 and earlier years), http://www.who.int/whosis. (Age-adjusted rates.)

**Figure 10.4**
**Country Differences in Female Heart Disease Mortality Rates, 1994–1996**

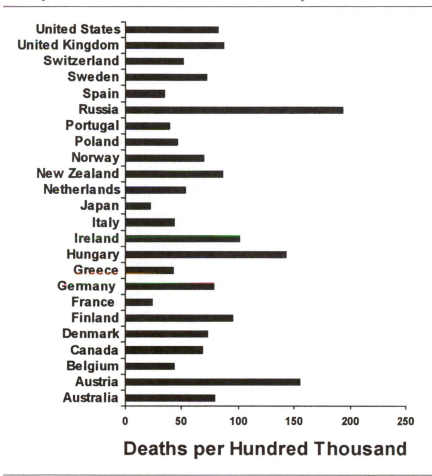

**Deaths per Hundred Thousand**

*Source:* World Health Organization, *World Health Statistics Annual* (Geneva, Switzerland: World Health Organization, 1996 and earlier years), http://www.who.int/whosis. (Age-adjusted rates.)

Europe. For example, the 1996 age-adjusted death rates from coronary heart disease among men equaled 149.8 deaths per hundred thousand in the United States, 159.9 in Sweden, 156.5 in Germany, and 185.9 in the United Kingdom. In contrast, the rates in Italy reached only 92.9, in France only 60.4, and in Spain only 78.2.

Declining mortality across high-income European nations has to some degree narrowed geographical differences. Much as it is today, heart disease mortality has historically been higher in northern European nations than southern European nations. Factors relating to diet, industrialization, and stress help explain the continued advantage of the southern European nations. However, since the northern European nations show faster declines in heart disease mortality than the southern European nations, the north-south differences in mortality have declined (but not disappeared) over the last several decades.[41]

In contrast, the former socialist nations of eastern Europe have extremely high rates of heart disease. Russia has age-adjusted rates of mortality from coronary heart disease in 1996 of 389.3 for men and 193.3 for women. These rates are more than two times higher than those in the United States and more than six to eight times higher than those in France. For the most part, nations of eastern Europe have experienced rising rather than falling heart disease mortality for the last several decades.[42] In the last few years, Poland has reversed the upward trend and enjoyed falling rates of mortality from coronary heart disease. Despite continued high levels of tobacco use, improvements in diet, alcohol use, and medical care, and adjustments to new economic and political institutions in other former communist nations could lead to improvements in rates of heart disease mortality.

Although coronary heart disease is viewed as a problem of affluent, industrialized societies, it is emerging as increasingly important in other parts of the world as well. Already the leading cause of death in the world, responsible for 6.3 million deaths across the globe in 1990, heart disease represents a major public health care problem in many low- and middle-income nations.[43] More worrisome, heart disease mortality rates are rising in these developing nations rather than falling as they are in developed nations. As newly rich societies usually experience an epidemic of coronary heart disease, the upward trend in the developing world today may duplicate the upward trend experienced in the developed world earlier in the twentieth century. It may also result from the Westernization of traditional diets, as households consume fewer fruits, grains, and vegetables and more high-calorie, refined carbohydrates.[44]

## THE CONTINUING HIGH INCIDENCE OF HEART DISEASE

Despite success in reducing heart disease mortality since the mid-1960s, several facts concern public health experts. Perhaps most important, the prevalence of heart disease has changed little in the last 10 years, even though death rates from heart disease continue to fall.[45] In the United States, for example, hospitalization rates for acute myocardial infarctions have declined only slightly for persons ages 45 to 64 and have actually risen for persons ages 65 and over. In southeastern New England from 1980 to 1991, fatal plus nonfatal coronary disease events remained stable because an increase in nonfatal hospitalization balanced a coinciding decrease in deaths.[46] Similarly, heart disease mortality in the Netherlands has decreased sharply, but rates of heart attacks—both fatal and nonfatal—have stayed constant.[47] Heart disease remains widespread but less often results in a fatality than in the past.

Continued progress against the incidence of heart disease requires something more than the ability to extend the lives of those who have the disease. It requires changes in the underlying presence of the disease. Otherwise, the increasingly large numbers of persons who have survived heart attacks and live with heart disease could overwhelm the health care system, produce greater levels of disability, and lower the quality of life of the population. The need to prevent new heart disease, not just treat existing heart disease, shows in other ways. Several risk factors, such as consumption of fat, hypertension, and cigarette smoking, have stopped declining at previous rates and foretell heart disease problems in decades to come.

Complacency about the problem may arise with declining deaths from heart disease and direct attention away from research and public health efforts that have had so much success in the past. Calls to action to prevent and treat heart disease thus continue. A government committee argues that we need a comprehensive approach to detecting and managing risk factors, increased attention to population subgroups at high risk, and mobilization of resources to implement these strategies.[48] Assuming that the battle against heart disease has already been won is a mistake. To the contrary, efforts to continue the battle—despite the successes in the last several decades—become all the more important in the twenty-first century.

# CHAPTER 11

# Looking Ahead

Vice President Dick Cheney announced on May 7, 2003, that he will run with President George W. Bush for reelection in 2004. Many wondered if his health would prevent him from doing so. As described in chapter 1, Cheney has had several heart attacks, heart bypass surgery, a stent placed in his coronary artery, an implanted pacemaker, and an implanted defibrillator. By age 62, he has battled heart disease for a quarter century. Yet he feels confident that despite his history of heart problems, medical care can keep him working at his time-consuming and stressful job for another four-year term. He states, "I've got a doc with me 24 hours a day who watches me very carefully. There's one outside there [the door] now. He's part of the entourage that supports me."[1] That quote reveals the confidence Cheney has in the ability of his doctors and the medical system more generally to deal with any further complications that might emerge.

There are good reasons for Cheney's confidence in medicine. The progress against heart disease in the past is undeniable, and continued progress in the future appears likely. Simple projections of heart disease mortality from the previous several decades to the next several decades imply a steady downward trend. If this occurs, heart disease may lose its position as the number-one killer of Americans, to be replaced by cancer, and average life expectancy will continue to rise. Are there reasons to suppose the trends will continue? At least for the near future, the answer appears to be yes. The forecast is not wholly positive, but sources of improvement should dominate in the future, as they have in the recent past.

This chapter briefly reviews recent and likely forthcoming developments in both medicine and lifestyle that may contribute to future progress against heart disease. In the area of medicine, experts are most optimistic. New knowledge and research advances have led scientists to expect new solutions to old problems—perhaps including innovative genetic therapies that will revolutionize treatment of heart disease and medicine more generally. In the area of lifestyle, changes will likely come more slowly. Modern medicine has done much to treat existing heart disease but has had less success getting people to change their lifestyles in ways that lower the likelihood of getting heart disease. Still, some reasons also exist to be optimistic about the ability to prevent heart disease through behavior rather than treatment.

## MEDICINE

Key innovations during the twentieth century include the development of

- a system of delivering emergency medical care—CPR, defibrillation, and advanced life support—to victims of cardiac arrest;
- widely used blood tests for cholesterol, high blood pressure, and diabetes that allow physicians to identify those at high risk for heart disease;
- diagnostic techniques such as the electrocardiogram and, more recently, cardiac catheterization and angiography;
- new medications to treat heart failure, angina, high blood pressure, and perhaps most important, high levels of blood cholesterol;
- less-invasive surgical procedures involving angioplasty and stents for coronary heart disease, and the implantation of pacemakers for heart arrhythmias; and
- procedures to make major surgeries for coronary artery bypass, valve repair and replacement, and heart transplantation safer and more effective.

Other developments, while not yet routinely used, appear promising. In terms of emergency medical care, efforts to make automatic external defibrillators available in places of business, public facilities, and the homes of heart patients will allow laypersons to use them when emergency personnel cannot. In terms of identifying risk factors, blood measures of inflammation, infectious bacteria, and blood clotting add to information obtained about the standard risk factors of cholesterol, high blood pressure, and diabetes. In terms of diagnosis, improvements in magnetic resonance imaging and computed tomography scanning can replace more invasive techniques.[2] In terms of treatment, medications may emerge that, like statins, directly deal with the inflammation and infections that create the conditions for the growth of plaque on the walls of the coronary arteries. In terms of surgery, use of minimally invasive surgery avoids many of the risks of open-heart surgery.[3]

## Future Developments

More advances continue to emerge. Over the last several years, the American Heart Association has listed the top 10 research advances made in the area of cardiovascular disease. These research advances will require much work and time before becoming widely used in clinical practice, but they have much promise. Listed here are several examples of the research advances from 2001 and 2002.[4]

First, several teams of researchers find that "transplanting cells from patients' own thigh muscles or bone marrow into dead or weakened heart tissue . . . may have the potential to replace scar with living tissue."[5] The procedure, used for patients who suffered a heart attack or heart failure, involves taking immature cells from the thigh that would otherwise become muscle cells, growing them into large quantities in the lab for three to four weeks, and injecting the cells into damaged areas of the heart. Causing no adverse effects, the cells show evidence that they take root and flourish in dead areas of the heart. They appear to help grow new muscle in the heart, although it is less clear if they make the heart beat more strongly.

Second, gene therapy can reduce angina. A naturally occurring protein called the vascular endothelial growth factor promotes the growth of new blood vessels. Studies find that injecting the gene for this protein into the heart reduces angina, increases the ability to exercise, and improves the flow of blood through the heart. The injections, made with a special catheter used to identify the parts of the heart lacking blood supply, appear not to cause any major complications in patients.

Third, robots can help perform a procedure to repair an opening between the heart's two upper chambers. Although traditionally done with open-heart surgery, the new procedure requires only four pencil-sized chest incisions. In making the incisions and repairs, the surgeon sits at a computer console a few yards away and uses robot-guided instruments. This minimally invasive surgery allows patients to leave the hospital and return to their normal activities much sooner than for major surgery. It also reduces the likelihood of complications resulting from opening the chest cavity, using a heart-lung machine, and stopping the heart.

Fourth, preliminary experiments with a new type of artificial heart reveal some benefits in prolonging the lives of heart failure patients who are too sick for a heart transplant. The battery-powered, two-pound device is implanted in the chest and mimics the function of the heart by circulating blood through the body (and improves greatly on the artificial heart tried unsuccessfully more than 20 years ago). Thus far, the new artificial heart extends lives by months rather than years and has been used only for patients unable to benefit from other treatments. Still, with improvements, it may eventually be used for healthier heart transplant patients without an available donor heart. Since millions of Americans have congestive heart failure and only two thousand donor hearts become available each year, the artificial heart can fill a crucial need.

Fifth, researchers have had success with a pump that takes over for just one of the heart's chambers. The left ventricular assist device boosts the pumping ability of the heart's most crucial chamber—the one that pumps blood through the aorta to the body. It thus complements the heart's function rather than replacing it altogether. Right now, the device serves as a short-term bridge for those waiting to receive a transplant. Perhaps it will become suitable for long-term use among those unable to receive a heart transplant.

Sixth, three newly discovered genes may explain why some families are prone to premature heart disease. By sifting through 62 genes of 352 people with coronary artery disease and 418 without, researchers identified distinct genes that regulate proteins for blood clotting and artery repair. Knowledge of the genetic components of heart disease may make it possible to identify the risk early in life and implement preventive measures.

The National Heart, Lung, and Blood Institute, as described in its strategic plan for the years 2003–2007, has the goal of exploiting these and other advances.[6] It proposes to support more research on how to safely and effectively apply gene therapy to humans, improve the outcome of heart transplants, increase the supply of donor organs, repair or replace damaged tissue with cell transplantation, and develop more effective surgical procedures and medication therapies.

Many of these advances help deal with coronary artery disease—the major source of premature mortality from heart disease. In addition, however, many focus on heart failure, a problem of growing importance as more persons survive to older ages. The long-term solution to heart failure—heart transplantation—is limited by available heart donors.[7] Artificial hearts, left ventricular assists device, cell transplantation, and genetic therapy can help deal with this problem.

### Regenerative Medicine

Those thinking about the more distant future suggest that regenerative medicine will revolutionize the treatment of disease. The term *regenerative medicine* refers to the attempt to create new forms of prevention and treatment that restore organs and tissues to their normal functions with natural human substances.[8] Cells have the genetic ability to use proteins and chemical signals to grow, restore, and repair themselves. Regenerative medicine aims to learn to use this ability in rebuilding damaged or worn-out tissues. The key is to discover the chemical signals that lead cells to create tissues or body parts. With knowledge of these natural signals, physicians can do more than correct problems in malfunctioning—they can make tissue as good as new. Rather than repairing old body parts, the aim would be to replace damaged parts with new parts. Implementation of this strategy can take at least three forms that show promise in the long term for dealing with heart disease and other maladies.[9]

First and most immediately, regenerative medicine seeks to use genes, proteins, and antibodies as medicines. For example, the body uses the vascular endothelial growth factor to help build blood vessels; experiments that have implanted the gene for this protein in damaged heart muscle prove promising. Some predict that the first of these treatments will be available soon and will make up half of all medications in 20 years.[10]

Second, regenerative medicine aims to create replacement body parts for those that no longer work. Rather than transplanting organs from other persons, it may be possible in the future to grow needed organs in the lab for transplantation. For example, it is now possible to build a new bladder, cartilage, and bone in the lab, and lab-grown blood vessels and heart valves may be on the way.

Third, regenerative medicine has the goal of using stem cells to rejuvenate tissue. Stem cells are the earliest cells to form after conception and the source of diverse types of tissues in the body. They thus carry the chemical codes that trigger the development of nerves, muscles, bones, and blood vessels and have the ability to repair or replace damaged tissue. Once scientists learn how these cells work, they hope to replace older tissue and organs with younger tissue and organs.[11] "Stem-cell research therefore holds great therapeutic potential and is relevant, not only to basic science researchers, but also to clinicians (who may need to consider such cell-based therapy in the future) and to their patients."[12] Stem cells may even produce a solution to aging: with aging viewed as the failure of stem cells to reproduce, replacing old stem cells with young stem cells may provide a solution to aging. One proponent states, "Humans may become immortal by the systematic replacement of stem cells."[13]

The full benefits of these innovations will likely not be realized for another 70 years or more.[14] Regenerative medicine remains largely a set of concepts now, but new discoveries have made the ideas behind it feasible. If the concepts reach fruition, physicians at the end of this century may look back at today's medicine as primitive, painful, and ineffective—much as we look back today at the failures and limitations of medicine early in the twentieth century.[15] Use of toxic chemicals to treat cancer, invasive surgery for heart problems, and medications obtained from plants may seem terribly crude compared with the use of the body's own chemical signals and proteins to repair, restore, and grow body tissue.

## MAKING THE CASE FOR REGENERATIVE MEDICINE

Dr. William Haseltine, chief executive officer of Human Genome Sciences, expects a revolution in medicine: "When we know, in effect, what our cells know, health care will be revolutionized, giving birth to regenerative medicine—ultimately including the prolongation of life by regenerating our aging bodies with younger cells."[16] Haseltine, who coined the term *regenerative medicine,* has himself done much to make the case for such a revolution. With a doctorate in biophysics from Harvard, he served as professor at the Dana-Farber Cancer Institute at Harvard Medical School, did pioneering research on cancer and AIDS, and has received more than 50 patents for his discoveries.[17] In 1992, he founded a company, Human Genome Sciences, to exploit the revolution in biomedicine and soon left academia (*genomics* refers to the science of identifying and analyzing the functions of genes). Since then, he has worked tirelessly for the company and for the ideas behind it. Besides his duties of raising funds for the company, leading its research and development projects, and promoting the goals of regenerative medicine, he founded and edits an online journal, *E-Biomed: A Journal of Regenerative Medicine,* to promote both the new field and his vision for the future.[18]

Haseltine and his company have the mission to develop products to prevent, cure, and treat diseases through the understanding of human genes.[19] Still a young company, Human Genome Sciences has discovered thousands of new genes, developed many patents, and brought several genetically based medicines to human trials. With this effort, Haseltine has become an entrepreneur as well as a scientist and geneticist. As a magazine profile states, "He's brilliant. He's swaggering. And he may soon be Genomics' first billionaire."[20] The goals of the company have not yet been realized, but Haseltine is confident in his predictions about how the understanding of genes and the human genome will transform medicine. He boldly states that once we "gain enough information to control the behavior of every cell in our bodies, . . . we will be able to heal any disease. We will be able to cause tissues to rebuild themselves."[21]

### Remaining Concerns

The expectations of continuing advances in medical treatment do not justify complacency. Many problems remain to be addressed. Realizing innovative goals requires increasing levels of funding for research on heart disease. However, even with increased funding and the development of new medical techniques, the high cost and inaccessibility of health care can limit use of the techniques. Issues of cost and access help explain the lower rate of decline in heart disease mortality among minority groups, low socioeconomic status groups, and rural residents and could become even more important in years to come. In addition, research in the past has focused primarily on men and ignored the high risks of heart disease among women; recent steps to require research on women and publicize the risks of heart disease for women need to continue to fully exploit the benefits of new techniques. In sum, medicine in the twenty-first century will need to apply knowledge of the importance of prevention and the benefits of treatment to a wider population.

Future advances must also do more to reduce the incidence of heart disease, which has not declined to the same extent as mortality.[22] As medicine becomes more effective in dealing with those having heart disease and the lifestyles that promote heart disease continue, treatment strategies may be overwhelmed by the growing number of patients. This emphasizes the need to improve lifestyle behaviors that contribute to heart disease as well as medical treatment for those with heart disease.


## LIFESTYLE

Progress in improving the diet, tobacco use, exercise, blood cholesterol, and blood pressure of the population contributed significantly to declining heart disease mortality. People once viewed red meat, eggs, and whole milk as essential to a healthy diet, cigarette smoking as fashionable, exercise as eccentric, and blood cholesterol and blood pressure as unimportant. Now, many have come to eat healthier fare, avoid cigarettes and secondhand smoke, participate in a wide variety of physical activities, and monitor their blood cholesterol and pressure. Such activities contributed to the drop in heart disease deaths since the 1960s.

However, the progress toward healthier lifestyles appears to have stalled by the 1990s.[23] Consumption of saturated fats has declined, but caloric intake and reliance on fast food prepared outside the home have grown. As a result, a disconcerting rise in overweight, obesity, and type 2 diabetes has occurred.[24] The steady decline in tobacco use from the mid-1960s to the late 1980s leveled off over the 1990s. The percentage of the population participating in moderate or vigorous physical activity has changed little in recent years. And progress in reducing blood cholesterol and hypertension has still left millions with dangerously high levels of both. Despite past progress, current fat consumption, smoking, inactivity, and high blood cholesterol and pressure remain above recommended levels.

The Healthy People 2010 Goals of the federal government aim to improve on the recent record, but it is less clear if the goals can be reached.[25] Consider the baseline measures of healthy lifestyles for the latest year available and the goals set by the government for 2010. While 28 percent of adults consumed two servings of fruit each day, the goal is to reach 75 percent. While 3 percent consumed three servings of vegetables, the goal is to reach 50 percent. While 36 percent did not exceed recommended levels of saturated fat, the goal is to reach 75 percent. While 76 percent did not smoke cigarettes, the goal is to reach 88 percent. While 32 percent of adults participated in moderate or vigorous exercise, the goal is to reach 50 percent. While 72 percent had normal blood pressure, the goal is to reach 84 percent. And while 79 percent had normal blood cholesterol levels, the goal is to reach 83 percent.

Substantial gaps remain between recent levels and many of the goals. Can the gaps be overcome to reach the goals? The answer is: Not without extraordinary effort. Part of the problem stems from the fact that early progress comes easier than later progress. Those prone to adopt healthy lifestyles will make changes after merely learning the facts about behavior and health. Others more resistant to change, less willing to sacrifice their desires for fatty food, relaxation, tobacco, and nicotine, and more willing to accept health risks from their lifestyle—these persons will not change easily. Future progress therefore appears more difficult than past progress.

Since Americans oppose trying to outlaw unhealthy lifestyles, efforts to improve behavioral choices have to rest on persuasion and incentives. Antismoking efforts provide perhaps the best model for using these means. Activities of the media, foundations, private organizations, and federal, state, and local governments to publicize the harm of smoking through research, educational, and advertising reflect efforts at persuasion. Legislation to prohibit advertising, raise taxes on cigarettes, implement comprehensive statewide antismoking ordinances, and ban smoking in public places reflects efforts to change incentives. The same strategies may have promise in other areas. To help improve diet and deal with the problem of obesity, some public health experts suggest imposing taxes on fatty foods and providing subsidies for fruit and vegetable purchases.[26] To improve blood pressure and associated maladies, federal officials have just recently called for a more aggressive approach to prevention, one that includes publicizing the seriousness of the problem and changing the levels that define high blood pressure.[27]

Efforts to prod people to act in ways that will improve their health in the long run—even if they require short-term sacrifice—will certainly continue. A national conference on cardiovascular disease recommends a renewed emphasis on primary-risk-factor prevention, detection, and management. By giving attention to all population subgroups, especially those at high risk, the strategy aims to mobilize diverse national and local resources toward improved heart health of the population.[28] There is no guarantee that efforts such as this will be successful, but they hold promise.

## COMPLEMENTARY AND ALTERNATIVE MEDICINE

Reflecting desires to prevent and treat heart disease and other health problems in nontraditional ways, a movement to use complementary and alternative medicine (CAM) has grown. CAM is defined as health care systems, practices, and products outside conventional medicine.[29] Complementary medicine is used in combination with conventional medicine, while alternative medicine is used in place of conventional medicine. The nonconventional options include

- systems that have developed in the West such as homeopathic and naturopathic medicine, and systems developed outside the West such as Chinese medicine;
- emphasis on the ability of the mind to influence the body through the use of meditation, prayer, humor, and patient support groups;
- biological-based therapies that rely on herbs, foods, vitamins, and other natural products;
- body-based methods such as chiropractic or osteopathic manipulation and massage; and
- energy therapies such as therapeutic touch and use of electromagnetic fields.

Advocates of CAM suggest that several of these approaches—herbal medicine, Chinese medicine, vitamins and supplements, special diets and foods, and yoga—help prevent and treat atherosclerosis.[30]

Scientific evidence has not established the effectiveness of most of these approaches, but this hasn't slowed the growth in their popularity. "In 1997 Americans made 627 million visits to practitioners of alternative medicine and spent $27 billion of their own money to pay for alternative therapies. In contrast, Americans made only 386 million visits to their family doctor."[31] Another statistic highlights the importance of CAM: "One out of every two persons in the United States between the ages of 35 and 49 years used at least one alternative therapy in 1997. That is a growth of 47.3 percent since 1990."[32] In 1998, the National Center for Complementary and Alternative Medicine was established by congressional mandate as part of the National Institutes of Health. Reflecting the popularity of CAM and the need for more knowledge about the practices, the center does scientific research, trains users, and disseminates authoritative information to the public.[33]

The ability of CAM to contribute in the past or the future to preventing or treating heart disease is, despite the testimonial of millions about its benefits, difficult to quantify. However, the emphasis of CAM on proper and healthy living through diet and behavior can, by improving lifestyles, help in making progress against heart disease.

## MORE LIVES TO BE SAVED

Although the signs are by no means all positive, the evidence of progress against heart disease in the past combined with new medical treatments and goals for behavior change suggest that the twenty-first century will see millions more lives saved. Some factors have slowed progress, and some groups have benefited less than others from the progress. And some of the grander claims of revolutionary advances in medical treatment involve more speculation than realization right now. Still, the evidence overall offers many reasons to be optimistic about the future battle against heart disease.

# Glossary

**ACE (angiotensin converting enzyme) inhibitor:** A type of medication that widens the arteries and makes it easier for the heart to pump blood by inhibiting the effects of angiotensin.

**ACTH:** Adrenocorticotropin hormone.

**acute:** Marked by sudden onset and short duration.

**adrenaline:** A hormone that excites the body and speeds the heartbeat.

**adrenocorticotropin hormone:** A hormone released by the pituitary gland in the stress-response process.

**AED:** Automated external defibrillator.

**age-adjusted mortality rate:** A rate that controls for differences in age makeup when comparing rates across diverse groups and populations.

**alpha-beta-blocker:** A type of medication that slows the heart and reduces blood pressure by moderating nerve impulses to blood vessels.

**American Heart Association:** A national organization that aims to reduce disability and death from cardiovascular disease.

**aneurysm:** Abnormal widening of an artery.

**angina pectoris:** A condition in which the heart muscle receives insufficient blood and produces chest pain.

**angiogram:** X-ray pictures of the heart or coronary arteries taken during an angiography.

**angiography:** A process using x-ray pictures to observe a special dye as it moves through the heart or coronary arteries; the dye is injected through a catheter.

**angioplasty:** Catheterization procedure used to widen narrowed arteries by inflating a small balloon (also called coronary angioplasty, balloon angioplasty, or percutaneous transluminal coronary angioplasty [PCTA]).

**angiotensin II:** A chemical in the body that causes blood vessels to constrict.

**angiotensin antagonist:** A type of medication that prevents narrowing of the blood vessels by shielding them from the effect of angiotensin II.

**anti-arrhythmia drug:** A type of medication used to treat a fast or irregular heart rhythm.

**anticoagulant:** A type of medication that prevents blood clotting.

**anti-hypertension drug:** A type of medication used to lower blood pressure.

**anxiety:** An abnormal or overwhelming sense of fear.

**aorta:** The largest artery in the body and attached directly to the left ventricle.

**arrhythmia:** Any form of abnormal rhythm of the heartbeat.

**artery:** A thick-walled vessel that carries blood from the heart to the body.

**artificial heart:** A mechanical device implanted in a patient to perform the pumping functions of the heart.

**artificial lung:** A machine that feeds oxygen to the blood and removes carbon dioxide from the blood by passing it through special mesh material (also called oxygenator).

**asystole:** The absence of electrical activity in the heart.

**atherectomy:** A procedure that uses a tiny, rotating, high-speed cutting drill to shave off plaque inside an artery.

**atherosclerosis:** The accumulation of plaque on the inside of artery walls, particularly the coronary arteries, and a major source of heart disease.

**atrial fibrillation:** An irregular and quivering beat of the upper chambers of the heart.

**atrium (pl. atria):** One of two upper chambers of the heart that receives blood from either the lungs (left) or the body (right).

**automated external defibrillator:** A portable electrical device that, by providing basic instructions, allows laypersons to defibrillate victims of cardiac arrest.

**automatic implantable defibrillator:** A surgically implanted electrical device to defibrillate victims of cardiac arrest.

**automatic nervous system:** The system that maintains functions of the body without a person's deliberate effort or control and consists of the sympathetic and parasympathetic nervous systems.

**beta-blocker:** A type of medication that moderates the release of adrenaline and is used to treat blood pressure and heart problems.

**bile acid sequestrant:** A type of medication used to lower blood cholesterol.

**blood pressure:** The force exerted on the walls of the blood vessels during the movement of blood pumped from the heart to the body (systolic) and during the movement of blood returning to the heart (diastolic).

**BMI:** Body-mass index.

**body-mass index:** The ratio of weight (in kilograms) to height (in meters squared); overweight is judged as a body-mass index of 25.0 or greater, and obesity as 30.0 or higher.

**bradycardia:** An abnormally slow heart rhythm.

**CABG:** Coronary artery bypass graft.

**calcification:** The formation of calcium deposits on tissue, particularly inside vessels walls and on heart valves.

**calcified:** Tissues containing calcium deposits.

**calcium channel blocker:** A type of medication that dilates blood vessels by interrupting the normal flow of calcium to cells.

**CAM:** Complementary and alternative medicine.

**carbon dioxide:** The gas created by cell metabolism, removed from the blood by the lungs, and expelled from the lungs during breathing.

**carbon monoxide:** A colorless, odorless gas that is toxic when breathed in large amounts.

**cardiac:** Relating to the heart.

**cardiac arrest:** The abrupt and immediate stoppage of the heart's ability to pump blood.

**cardiac catheterization:** The insertion of a catheter through blood vessels to the heart and coronary arteries for the purpose of diagnosing and treating heart problems.

**cardiac enzyme:** A substance that initiates or speeds up chemical reactions and can indicate the occurrence of a heart attack.

**cardiology:** The study of the heart, its functions, and its diseases.

**cardiomyopathy:** A disease of the heart muscle that weakens its pumping ability.

**cardiopulmonary resuscitation:** A procedure designed to restore normal breathing and circulate blood through the body.

**cardiovascular:** Relating to the heart and system of blood vessels.

**cardioversion:** A process that converts an ineffective cardiac rhythm into a normal, spontaneous rhythm.

**cardioverter-defibrillator:** An implanted electrical device that uses electrical discharges to correct fibrillation of the heart.

**catheter:** A long thin tube used in catheterization.

**CCU:** Coronary care unit.

**Centers for Disease Control and Prevention:** The lead federal agency for protecting the health and safety of Americans.

**cholesterol:** A type of fat or lipid that circulates through the blood stream for use by the body but which also tends to accumulate on vessel walls.

**chronic:** Marked by long duration or frequent recurrence.

**clot:** A clump of blood cells that can stop the flow of blood in an injury but can also form inside an artery and cause a heart attack (also called thrombus).

**clot-busting (or clot-dissolving) drug:** A drug used to break up blood clots in the coronary arteries during a heart attack (also called thrombolytic agent).

**complementary and alternative medicine:** Health care systems, practices, and products outside conventional medicine.

**computed tomography:** The use of a rotating x-ray tube to provide a three-dimensional picture of the heart and other body organs.

**congenital malformation:** An abnormality in the structure and functioning of a body part present at birth.

**congestive heart failure:** The accumulation of fluid in the veins and parts of the body as a result of the heart's weakened ability to pump.

**coronary artery:** A blood vessel that brings oxygen-rich blood to the heart muscle.

**coronary artery bypass graft:** A new vessel attached to bypass a blockage in the coronary arteries and restore blood flow to the heart muscle.

**coronary artery bypass graft surgery:** A procedure to attach new vessels that bypass blockages in the coronary arteries and restore blood flow to the heart muscle.

**coronary artery (or coronary heart) disease:** The narrowing of a coronary artery that restricts the flow of blood to the heart muscle.

**coronary care unit:** A specialized hospital facility designed to monitor, treat, and care for coronary patients.

**coronary spasm:** An abnormal, intermittent constricting of a coronary artery.

**corticotrophin-releasing hormone:** A hormone released by the hypothalamus in the stress-response process.

**cortisol:** A hormone released by the adrenal glands in the stress-response process.

**CPR:** Cardiopulmonary resuscitation.

**C-reactive protein:** A protein that increases with inflammation and can serve as a marker of the swelling of vessels.

**CRH:** Corticotrophin-releasing hormone.

**CT (or CAT):** Computed tomography.

**defibrillation:** A procedure to deliver an electrical shock to the heart to restore its normal rhythm.

**defibrillator:** A device used to deliver an electrical shock to the heart from either outside (external) or inside (internal) the body.

**depression:** In clinical terms, a state characterized by extreme sadness, hopelessness, inactivity, and suicidal thoughts.

**diabetes:** A disease caused by the abnormal production or use of insulin, a hormone used to turn sugar and other foods into energy.

**diastole:** The part of the heartbeat when the heart is relaxing and filling with blood from the veins.

**diastolic:** The state of the heart when it is relaxing and receiving blood; also, the second measure of blood pressure.

**digitalis:** A medication used to treat heart failure by strengthening the pumping of the heart.

**dilated cardiomyopathy:** A weakening of the heart muscle that causes the heart chambers to enlarge.

**diuretic:** A type of medication that promotes the removal of water from the blood and body.

**dropsy:** A term used in the past to refer to heart failure.

**ECG (or EKG):** Electrocardiogram.

**echocardiography:** The use of echoed sound waves to observe the heart in motion.

**ejection fraction:** The percentage of blood ejected from the left ventricle (normal percentage is about 60 percent).

**electrocardiogram:** A graphical record of electrical activity of the heart.

**electrode:** A tiny sensor of electrical currents.

**electronic beam computed tomography:** A special form of computed tomography that detects abnormal calcification in the coronary arteries and elsewhere in the body (also called ultrafast CT).

**embolism:** A breakage of a blood clot that travels through the blood stream and lodges in another part of the blood vessel system.

**emergency medical technician:** Medical technician who is specially trained to provide basic emergency life support.

**EMT:** Emergency medical technician.

**epidemic:** The sudden outbreak and rapid spread of a disease (or form of behavior).

**epidemiological:** Relating to epidemiology, the branch of medical science concerned with the incidence and distribution of diseases in populations.

**epinephrine:** A hormone released by the adrenal glands in the stress-response process.

**estrogen:** Female sex hormone.

**estrogen replacement therapy:** The use of medication containing estrogen and other products to deal with symptoms of menopause and, ideally, reduce the risk of heart disease and osteoporosis.

**exercise stress test:** An electrocardiogram obtained during physical activity that raises the heartbeat (also called stress test).

**fatty acid:** A chemical that occurs naturally in the form of essential fats and oils.

**fiber:** Indigestible material in human food.

**fibrate:** A type of medication used to lower triglycerides and cholesterol.

**fibrillation:** An irregular and quivering beat of the heart.

**fibrinogen:** A protein in blood used in the formation of blood clots.

**gender:** Refers in this context to learned psychological, social, and cultural sources of differences between men and women (compare *sex*).

**genome:** The complete set of chromosomes and genes of an organism.

**genomics:** The science of identifying and analyzing the functions of specific genes.

**glucose:** The usual form in which carbohydrates are absorbed by the body.

**graft:** A surgical implant of living tissue.

**HDL:** High-density lipoprotein.

**heart attack:** The death or damage of heart tissue that results from the failure of blood to reach the heart muscle (more precisely called myocardial infarction).

**heart block:** A slowed heart rhythm due to the failure of electrical impulses to reach the lower chambers of the heart.

**heart disease:** An abnormal or malfunctioning condition of the heart and circulation, including problems with the heart muscle, valves, rhythm, flow of blood to the heart, and circulation of blood from the heart to the body.

**heart failure:** Symptoms caused by diseases in which the heart is unable to pump enough blood to meet the body's requirements.

**heart-lung machine:** A mechanical pump that circulates and provides oxygen to the blood during heart surgery (also called pump oxygenator).

**heart transplant surgery:** A procedure to replace a defective heart in one patient with the healthy heart of a recently deceased person.

**heart valve:** The thin heart tissue between chambers that causes the blood to be pumped in one direction (includes tricuspid, mitral, pulmonary, and aortic valves).

**heart valve surgery:** A procedure to repair or replace a defective heart valve.

**Heimlich maneuver:** The abrupt use of pressure on the upper abdomen to expel a foreign object obstructing air flow to the lungs from the throat or larynx (voice box).

**heparin:** A medication used to prevent blood clotting.

**high blood pressure drug:** A type of medication used to lower blood pressure.

**high-density lipoprotein:** A substance that transports cholesterol to the liver where it is broken down and removed from the body and, in so doing, prevents the accumulation of cholesterol along vessel walls.

**HMG-CoA reductase:** The main cholesterol-lowering agent in statins.

**Holter monitor:** A device that continuously records electrical activity of the heart for future analysis.

**hormone:** A product of the body that stimulates cell activity and performs other crucial functions.

**HPA axis:** Hypothalamic-pituitary-adrenal axis.

**hypertension:** High blood pressure.

**hypertrophic cardiomyopathy:** A heart muscle that becomes thicker and stiffer than normal.

**hypothalamic-pituitary-adrenal axis:** The process of hormone release triggered by the nervous system in response to stress.

**immune system:** Protects the body from foreign substances, cells, and tissues.

**insulin:** A hormone used by the body to process carbohydrates.

**intravenous:** The delivery of liquids, nutrients, medications, and other products to the body through a tube inserted into a vein.

**intubation:** The insertion of a tube down the throat to deliver oxygen to the lungs and aid victims of cardiac arrest in breathing.

**ischemia:** Decreased blood flow to an organ such as the heart, usually due to narrowing or blockage of an artery.

**ischemic heart disease:** The insufficiency of blood to the heart, usually from narrowing of the coronary arteries.

**IV:** Intravenous.

**laser ablation:** A procedure that uses a tiny laser beam to vaporize plaque along an artery wall.

**LDL:** Low-density lipoprotein.

**left ventricular assist device:** A mechanical device implanted in a patient to replace the pumping function of the left ventricle but not the other chambers.

**lipid:** A substance such as cholesterol or triglyceride that is needed by the body and circulates in the blood.

**lipoprotein:** A substance that carries cholesterol and other materials in the blood.

**lipoprotein(a):** A blood particle that helps repair torn blood vessels but also can promote blood clots in the coronary arteries.

**long QT syndrome:** An inherited condition that leads to cardiac arrest and sudden death often in children, youth, and young people.

**low-density lipoprotein:** A substance that transports cholesterol to sites throughout the body for use by cells but also contributes to the accumulation of cholesterol along vessel walls.

**magnetic resonance imaging:** The use of magnetic field and radio waves to obtain detailed images of the heart and other parts of the body.

**menopause:** Physical changes that occur to women, usually during ages 40 to 50, associated with the end of menstruation and the ability to conceive.

**metabolic:** Relating to metabolism, or the changes that occur in the body and cells when transforming substances into energy.

**metabolic syndrome:** The occurrence of multiple abnormalities associated with increased blood sugar, blood lipids, and blood pressure during aging (also called syndrome X).

**minimally invasive bypass surgery:** A form of bypass surgery done without opening the chest cavity, stopping the heart, or using a pump oxygenator.

**monounsaturated fat:** A type of unsaturated fat found, for example, in olive and peanut oil.

**mortality rate:** The number of deaths in a population or group divided by the size of the population or group.

**MRI:** Magnetic resonance imaging.

**myocardial infarction:** The death or damage of heart tissue that results from the failure of blood to reach the heart muscle (also called heart attack).

**myocardium:** Muscular tissue of the heart.

**National Heart, Lung, and Blood Institute:** Part of the National Institutes of Health, it supports research on understanding the causes of diseases of the heart, lung, and blood and on preventing these diseases.

**National Institutes of Health:** A government organization that sponsors government-supported medical and behavioral research on health.

**nicotine:** The chemical component of tobacco that has the effect of stimulating the mind and relaxing the muscles but also leads to addiction.

**nicotinic acid:** A medication used to lower cholesterol.

**norepinephrine:** A hormone released by the adrenal glands in the stress-response process.

**nuclear imaging technique:** A procedure used to observe the movement of a radioactive substance through the heart, vessels, and other parts of the body.

**obesity:** A condition characterized by excessive fat and body weight.

**omega-3 fatty acid:** Found in fish and fish oils, a substance that has beneficial effects for the heart.

**osteoporosis:** A decrease in bone mass that produces fragility and curvature of the spine.

**oxidized LDL cholesterol:** A form of LDL cholesterol that combines with oxygen and contributes to atherosclerosis.

**oxygenator:** A machine that feeds oxygen to the blood and removes carbon dioxide from the blood by passing it through special mesh material (also called artificial lung).

**pacemaker:** An electrical device with electrodes implanted in the heart to regulate the heart rhythm by emitting electrical discharges.

**paramedic:** A specially trained medical technician who provides advanced emergency life support.

**parasympathetic nervous system:** The nervous system that causes slowing of body functions and the heartbeat.

**PCTA:** Percutaneous transluminal coronary angioplasty.

**percutaneous transluminal coronary angioplasty:** The formal name for angioplasty.

**perfusion scan:** A nuclear imaging technique used to determine damage to heart tissue.

**phytochemical:** A micronutrient such as plant sterol and stanol that shows promise for reducing the risk of atherosclerosis.

**plaque:** A material consisting of cholesterol, calcium, immune cells, and other substances that tends to accumulate along the walls of the blood vessels in atherosclerosis.

**platelets:** Small blood cells used in the formation of blood clots.

**polyunsaturated fat:** A type of unsaturated fat found, for example, in corn and soybean oil.

**premature ventricular contraction:** An extra heartbeat that arises from the contraction of the lower chambers of the heart.

**primary prevention:** The effort to prevent heart disease among persons without the disease or symptoms of the disease.

**psychosocial:** Relating to both psychological and social factors.

**pulmonary artery:** The artery that carries unoxygenated blood from the heart to the lungs.

**pulmonary vein:** The vein that carries oxygenated blood from the lungs to the heart.

**pump oxygenator:** A mechanical pump that circulates and provides oxygen to the blood during heart surgery (also called heart-lung machine).

**radioactive:** Characteristic of substances that give off radiant energy and can be detected by special equipment.

**radioisotope:** A radioactive substance used in nuclear scanning.

**radionuclide ventriculography:** A nuclear imaging technique that observes and measures ejection of blood from the left ventricle of the heart.

**regenerative medicine:** The use of natural substances such as human cells, genetics, and chemicals to restore or regenerate damaged or worn-out tissues and organs.

**revascularization:** A surgical procedure such as angioplasty or coronary artery bypass graft that provides new or additional blood supply to the heart and other body parts.

**SADS:** Sudden arrhythmia death syndrome.

**saturated fat:** A type of fat found usually in foods from animals such as meat and diary products.

**secondary prevention:** The effort to prevent heart disease from worsening among persons already with the disease.

**sedentary:** Term used to describe a person who engages in little or no physical activity.

**selective serotonin reuptake inhibitor:** A type of medication used to treat depression.

**sex:** Refers in this context to biological sources of differences between men and women (compare *gender*).

**socioeconomic status:** One's position in society based on education, prestige, and income.

**sodium:** A mineral essential for life and contained in table salt.

**statin:** A type of medication used to lower blood cholesterol.

**stem cell:** A type of cell that is the first to form after conception and is the source of diverse types of tissues throughout the body.

**stent:** A small wire mesh tube (sometimes coated with a drug) that is placed in an artery after an angioplasty to prevent the widened artery from collapsing.

**stress:** The physical, psychological, and emotional response to situations viewed as problematic or threatening to one's health or psychological well-being.

**stress test:** An electrocardiogram obtained during increasing physical activity that raises the heartbeat (also called exercise stress test).

**sudden arrhythmia death syndrome:** An inherited condition that results in sudden death in children, youth, and young people.

**sympathetic nervous system:** The nervous system that causes excitement or arousal of the body and speeds the heartbeat.

**Syndrome X:** The occurrence of multiple abnormalities associated with increased blood sugar, blood lipids, and blood pressure during aging (also called metabolic syndrome).

**systolic:** The state of the heart when it is contracting and pumping blood out; also the first measure of blood pressure.

**tachycardia:** An abnormally fast heart rhythm.

**tar:** Particles contained in tobacco smoke that are harmful to the heart and other parts of the body.

**testosterone:** Male sex hormone.

**thoracic:** Relating to the chest-cavity area of the upper body.

**thrombolytic agent:** A type of medication used to break up blood clots in the coronary arteries during a heart attack (also called clot-busting or clot-dissolving drug).

**thrombosis:** The formation of a clot or thrombus.

**thrombus:** A clot or clump of blood cells that can stop the flow of blood in an injury but that can also form inside an artery and cause a heart attack.

**triglyceride:** A lipid used by the body as a source of energy.

**type 2 diabetes:** A form of diabetes involving lessening amounts of insulin or lessening effectiveness of insulin (also called adult-onset diabetes).

**Type A behavior:** Coronary-prone behavior marked by a sense of time urgency and free-floating hostility.

**Type B behavior:** The absence of Type A behavior and its associated consequence for developing coronary heart disease.

**ultrafast CT:** A special form of computed tomography that detects abnormal calcification in the coronary arteries and elsewhere in the body (also called electronic beam computed tomography).

**unsaturated fat:** A type of fat obtained from vegetable food products, it includes monounsaturated and polyunsaturated fats.

**U.S. Food and Drug Administration:** The government agency responsible for reviewing clinical research and regulating food and medical products to ensure they are safe.

**valvular regurgitation:** The ineffective closing of the heart valves that allows blood to flow back.

**valvular stenosis:** The narrowing of the heart valves that prevents blood from flowing fully from one chamber to the next.

**vascular:** Relating to the blood vessels.

**vascular endothelial growth factor:** A naturally occurring protein that can be used through genetic engineering to help grow new vessels in the heart.

**vasodilator:** A type of medication that widens the blood vessels.

**vein:** A thin-walled vessel that carries blood from the body back to the heart.

**ventricle:** One of two lower chambers of the heart that sends blood to either the lungs (right ventricle) or the body (left ventricle).

**ventricular fibrillation:** An irregular and quivering beat of the lower chambers of the heart.

**warfarin:** A blood-thinning medication that is useful for persons with heart failure.

**x-ray:** A radiation wave capable of penetrating through dense materials and used for pictures of the heart and other body parts.

# Notes

## CHAPTER 1: COUNTING THE LIVES SAVED

1. Cable News Network, "Cheney's History of Heart Problems," June 29, 2001, http://www.cnn.com/2000/HEALTH/06/29/cheney.chronology.

2. Cable News Network, "Letterman Expected to Fully Recover from Heart Surgery," January 14, 2000, http://www.cnn.com/2000/SHOWBIZ/TV/01/15/letterman.heart.

3. Tom Monte and Ilene Pritikin, *Pritikin: The Man Who Healed America's Heart* (Emmaus, Penn.: Rodale Press, 1997).

4. U.S. Department of Health and Human Services, "HHS Study Finds Life Expectancy in the U.S. Rose to 77.2 Years in 2001," News Release, March 14, 2003, http://www.hhs.gov/news/press/2003pres/20030314a.html.

5. National Heart, Lung, and Blood Institute, "Morbidity and Mortality: 2002 Chart Book on Cardiovascular, Lung, and Blood Diseases," October 20, 2002, http://www.nhlbi.nih.gov/resources/docs/02-chtbk.pdf.

6. National Heart, Lung, and Blood Institute, "2002 Chart Book," p. 9.

7. Morris Notelovitz and Diana Tonnessen, *The Essential Heart Book for Women* (New York: St. Martin's Press, 1996), p. 2.

8. National Heart, Lung, and Blood Institute, "2002 Chart Book," p. 17.

9. National Heart, Lung, and Blood Institute, "2002 Chart Book," p. 32.

10. R. A. Stallones, "The Rise and Fall of Ischemic Heart Disease," *Scientific American* 243 (November 1980): 43–50.

11. E. Braunwald, "Cardiovascular Medicine at the Turn of the Millennium: Triumphs, Concerns, and Opportunities," *New England Journal of Medicine* 337 (1997): 1360–69.

12. M. S. Brown and J. L. Goldstein, "Heart Attacks: Gone with the Century?" *Science*, May 3, 1996, p. 629.

13. Brown and Goldstein, "Heart Attacks," p. 630.

14. R. J. Lefkowitz and J. T. Willerson, "Prospects for Cardiovascular Research," *Journal of the American Medical Association* 285 (2001): 581–87.

15. Braunwald, "Cardiovascular Medicine."

16. Braunwald, "Cardiovascular Medicine."

17. J. I. Breslow, "Battling Heart Disease," *Science,* July 5, 1996, pp. 15–18.

18. C. J. Murray and A. D. Lopez, "Alternative Projections of Mortality and Disability by Cause 1990–2020: Global Burden of Disease Study," *Lancet* 349 (1997): 1498–1504.

19. Braunwald, "Cardiovascular Medicine."

20. Steven Lehrer, *Explorers of the Body* (Garden City, N.Y.: Doubleday, 1979), pp. 4–5.

21. P. E. Baldry, *The Battle against Heart Disease* (Cambridge, England: Cambridge University Press, 1971), pp. 5–6.

22. Lehrer, *Explorers of the Body,* pp. 5–6.

23. Bernard J. Gersh, ed., *Mayo Clinic Heart Book,* 2nd ed. (New York: William Morrow, 2000), pp. 44–45.

24. Quoted in Lehrer, *Explorers of the Body,* p. 10.

25. Quoted in Baldry, *Battle against Heart Disease,* p. 19.

26. Brown and Goldstein, "Heart Attacks," pp. 629–30.

27. R. M. Lawn, "Lipoprotein(a) in Heart Disease," *Scientific American* 266 (June 1992): 54–60.

28. R. Ross, "Atherosclerosis: An Inflammatory Disease," *New England Journal of Medicine* 340 (1999): 115–26.

29. Paul W. Ewald, *Plague Time: How Stealth Infections Cause Cancers, Heart Disease, and Other Deadly Ailments* (New York: Free Press, 2000), p. 109.

30. F. J. Nieto, "Cardiovascular Disease and Risk Factor Epidemiology: A Look Back at the Epidemic of the 20th Century," *American Journal of Public Health* 89 (March 1999): 292–94.

31. J. Danesh, R. Collins, and R. Peto, "Chronic Infections and Coronary Heart Disease: Is There a Link?" *Lancet* 350 (1997): 430–36.

32. Ewald, *Plague Time,* pp. 107–15.

33. Braunwald, "Cardiovascular Medicine."

34. K. Kuulasmaa et al., "Estimation of Contribution of Changes in Classic Risk Factors to Trends in Coronary-Event Rates across the WHO MONICA Project Populations," *Lancet* 355 (2000): 675–87.

35. P. Magnus and R. Beaglehole, "The Real Contribution of the Major Risk Factors to the Coronary Epidemics: Time to End the 'Only-50%' Myth," *Archives of Internal Medicine* 161 (2001): 2657–60.

36. K. Haskin, "Bates Dies of Enlarged Heart," *Topeka Capital Journal,* August 3, 2000, http://cjonline.com/stories/080300/spo_bates.shtml.

37. American Heart Association, "Statistical Fact Sheet—Populations: Youth and Cardiovascular Diseases," http://www.americanheart.org/presenter.jhtml?identifier=2011 (accessed May 2003).

38. American Heart Association, *Heart Disease and Stroke Statistics: 2003 Update,* http://www.americanheart.org/presenter.jhtml?identifier=1928 (accessed May 2003), pp. 4, 12; American Heart Association, "Statistical Fact Sheet—Populations:

Youth and Cardiovascular Diseases"; Kathleen Berra et al., *Heart Attack: Advice for Patients by Patients* (New Haven, Conn.: Yale University Press, 2002), pp. 94–101.

39. J. L. Thomas and P. A. Braus, "Coronary Artery Disease in Women: A Historical Perspective," *Archives of Internal Medicine* 158 (1998): 333–37.

## CHAPTER 2: EMERGENCY LIFESAVING TREATMENT

1. The story of John Colven appears in Mickey S. Eisenberg, *Life in the Balance: Emergency Medicine and the Quest to Reverse Sudden Death* (New York: Oxford University Press, 1997), pp. 23–29.

2. R. G. Sachs and J. Kerwin, "Automated External Defibrillators and Sudden Cardiac Arrest," *New Jersey Medicine* 98 (April 1998): 39.

3. K. Kennedy and R. Deitsch, eds., "Scorecard: For the Record," *Sports Illustrated*, January 20, 2003, p. 20.

4. Eisenberg, *Life in the Balance*, p. x.

5. L. Goldman and E. F. Cook, "Reasons for the Decline in Coronary Heart Disease Mortality: Medical Interventions versus Life-Style Changes," in *Trends in Coronary Heart Disease: The Influence of Medical Care*, ed. Millicent W. Higgins and Russell V. Luepker (New York: Oxford University Press, 1988), pp. 67–75.

6. Stefan Timmermans, *Sudden Death and the Myth of CPR* (Philadelphia: Temple University Press, 1999), pp. 1–10.

7. R. J. Myerburg et al., "Definitions and Epidemiology of Sudden Cardiac Death," in *Fighting Sudden Cardiac Death: A Worldwide Challenge*, ed. Etienne Aliot, Jacques Clementy, and Eric N. Prystowsky (Armonk, N.Y.: Futura, 2000), p. 4.

8. L. F. Fallin, "Cardiopulmonary Resuscitation (CPR)," *Gale Encyclopedia of Medicine*, vol. 2, ed., Jacqueline L. Longe (Farmington Hills, Mich.: Gale Group, 2002), pp. 661–65.

9. G. Ewy, "Cardiopulmonary Resuscitation: Strengthening the Links in the Chain of Survival," *New England Journal of Medicine* 342 (2000): 1599–1601.

10. R. M. Robertson, "Sudden Death from Cardiac Arrest: Improving the Odds," *New England Journal of Medicine* 343 (2000): 1259.

11. R. O. Cummins et al., "Improving Survival from Sudden Cardiac Arrest: The 'Chain of Survival' Concept," American Heart Association, http://216.185.112.41/Science/ISFSCAstatement.htm.

12. J. M. Fisher, "The Resuscitation Greats: The Earliest Records," *Resuscitation* 44 (April 2000): 79–80.

13. Quoted in Fisher, "Resuscitation Greats," p. 80.

14. 1 Kings 17:17.

15. 2 Kings 4:32–35.

16. Fallin, "Cardiopulmonary Resuscitation."

17. Ewy, "Cardiopulmonary Resuscitation."

18. A. Hallstrom et al., "Cardiopulmonary Resuscitation by Chest Compression Alone or with Mouth-to-Mouth Ventilation," *New England Journal of Medicine* 342 (2000): 1546–53.

19. Robertson, "Sudden Death from Cardiac Arrest," p. 1259.

20. Robertson, "Sudden Death from Cardiac Arrest."

21. J. W. Gundry et al., "Comparison of Naïve Sixth-Grade Children with Trained Professionals in the Use of an Automated External Defibrillator," *Circulation* 100 (1999): 1703–7.

22. American Heart Association, "Questions and Answers about AEDs," http://216.185.112.41/cpr_aed/cpr_aed_menu.htm (accessed October 2002).

23. M. S. Eisenberg, "Is It Time for Over-the-Counter Defibrillators?" *Journal of the American Medical Association* 284 (2000): 1435–38.

24. Cummins et al., "Improving Survival," p. 13.

25. Goldman and Cook, "Reasons for the Decline," pp. 68–69.

26. M. McCarthy, "Looking After Your Neighbors Seattle-Style," *Lancet* 351 (1998): 732.

27. M. S. Eisenberg, "Resuscitation Greats: Leonard Cobb and Medic One," *Resuscitation* 54 (July 2002): 5–9.

28. M. S. Eisenberg, quoted in McCarthy, "Looking After Your Neighbors," p. 732.

29. Eisenberg, "Resuscitation Greats," p. 7.

30. Eisenberg, "Resuscitation Greats," p. 8.

31. Eisenberg, *Life in the Balance*, pp. 60–61.

32. Timmermans, *Sudden Death and the Myth of CPR*, pp. 46–47.

33. P. E. Baldry, *The Battle against Heart Disease* (Cambridge, England: Cambridge University Press, 1971), p. 132.

34. Eisenberg, *Life in the Balance*, p. 195.

35. Eisenberg, *Life in the Balance*, pp. 196–99.

36. Eisenberg, *Life in the Balance*, pp. 203–18.

37. Myerburg et al., "Definitions and Epidemiology," p. 4.

38. Myerburg et al., "Definitions and Epidemiology," p. 5.

39. McCarthy, "Looking After Your Neighbors," p. 732.

40. T. Parker-Pope, "A Poor Track Record May Force Changes in How We Do CPR," *New York Times*, March 31, 2000, sec. B, p. 1, col. 1.

41. Robertson, "Sudden Death from Cardiac Arrest," p. 1259.

42. Eisenberg, "Is It Time for Over-the-Counter Defibrillators?" p. 1438.

43. Ewy, "Cardiopulmonary Resuscitation."

44. Cummins et al., "Improving Survival from Sudden Cardiac Arrest," p. 15.

45. Goldman and Cook, "Reasons for the Decline," pp. 68–69.

46. Timmermans, *Sudden Death and the Myth of CPR*, pp. 56–89.

47. M. S. Eisenberg and T. J. Mengert, "Cardiac Resuscitation," *New England Journal of Medicine* 344 (2001): 1304–13.

48. Eisenberg, *Life in the Balance*, pp. 251–52.

## CHAPTER 3: DIAGNOSING HEART DISEASE

1. Clarence G. Lasby, *Eisenhower's Heart Attack: How Ike Beat Heart Disease and Held On to the Presidency* (Lawrence: University Press of Kansas, 1997).

2. G. Ertl, "Book Review: Difficult Cardiology III," *New England Journal of Medicine* 338 (1998): 1704–5.

3. Many sources offer overviews of common cardiology tests. The material to follow relies on several such sources: American Heart Association, *Your Heart: An Owner's Manual* (Englewood Cliffs, N.J.: Prentice-Hall, 1995); C. Bianco, "How Diagnosing Heart Disease Works," How Stuff Works, http://www.howstuffworks.com/heart-diagnosis.htm (accessed January 2003); Bernard J. Gersh, ed., *Mayo Clinic Heart Book*, 2nd ed. (New York: William Morrow, 2000);

Leonard S. Lilly, ed., *Pathophysiology of Heart Disease* (Baltimore, Md.: Lippincott, Williams, and Wilkins, 2003); Merck, *Diagnosis of Heart Disease, The Merck Manual: Home Edition*, http://www.merck.com/pubs/mmanual_home/sec3/15.htm (accessed April 2003); Texas Heart Institute, *Heart Owner's Manual* (New York: Wiley, 1996), pp. 329–35; and Adam D. Timmons, Anthony W. Nathan, and Ian D. Sullivan, *Essential Cardiology*, Oxford: Blackwell Science, 1997).

4. The guidelines come from the National Cholesterol Education Program (revised 2001). See American Heart Association, "Cholesterol Levels: AHA Recommendations," http://www.americanheart.org/presenter.jhtml?identifier = 4500 (accessed April 2003).

5. P. M. Ridker, "Comparison of C-Reactive Protein and Low-Density Lipoprotein Cholesterol Levels in the Prediction of First Cardiovascular Events," *New England Journal of Medicine* 347 (2002): 1557.

6. American Heart Association, "Inflammation, Heart Disease and Strokes: The Role of C-Reactive Protein," http://www.americanheart.org/presenter. jhtml?identifier = 4648 (accessed April 2003).

7. J. Mercola, "Iron Overload Disorder Common and Increases Risk for Heart Attacks," http://www.mercola.com/1999/archive/iron_overload_disorder_ increases_heart_attack_risk.htm (accessed April 2003).

8. American Heart Association, "Iron and Heart Disease," http:// www.americanheart.org/presenter.jhtml?identifier = 4604 (accessed April 2003).

9. American Heart Association, "Cholesterol Levels: AHA Recommendations."

10. R. Volker, "Preventing CHD in Children," *Journal of the American Medical Association* 280 (1998): 2067.

11. A. M. Garber et al., "Cholesterol Screening in Asymptomatic Adults, Revisited," *Annals of Internal Medicine* 124 (March 1996): 518–31.

12. W. E. Leery, "Doctors' Group Recommends Reducing Cholesterol Checks," *New York Times*, March 1, 1996, sec. A, p. 18, col. 1.

13. T. B. Newman, W. S. Browner, and S. B. Hulley, "The Case against Childhood Cholesterol Screening," *Journal of the American Medical Association* 264 (1990): 3039–43.

14. American Heart Association, "Cholesterol Screening in Asymptomatic Adults," http://www.americanheart.org/presenter.jhtml?identifier = 429 (accessed April 2003).

15. J. Stamler, "Relationship of Baseline Serum Cholesterol Levels in 3 Large Cohorts of Younger Men to Long-Term Coronary, Cardiovascular, and All-Cause Mortality and to Longevity," *Journal of the American Medical Association* 284 (2000): 311–18.

16. J. P. Strong, "Prevalence and Extent of Atherosclerosis in Adolescents and Young Adults," *Journal of the American Medical Association* 281 (1999): 727–35.

17. W. Bao et al., "Longitudinal Changes in Cardiovascular Risk from Childhood to Young Adulthood in Offspring of Parents with Coronary Artery Disease: The Bogalusa Heart Study." *Journal of the American Medical Association* 278 (1997): 1749–54.

18. H. Lagström et al., "Modifying Coronary Heart Disease Risk Factors in Children: Is It Ever Too Early to Start?" *Journal of the American Medical Association* 279 (1998): 1261–62.

19. G. Kolata, "Cheaper Body Scans Spread, Despite Doubts," *New York Times*, May 27, 2002, sec. A, p. 1, col. 4.

20. Kolata, "Cheaper Body Scans Spread."

21. M. Mitka, "Imaging to Diagnose Cardiovascular Disease," *Journal of the American Medical Association* 289 (2003): 288–89.

22. Lilly, *Pathophysiology of Heart Disease*, p. 71.

23. P. E. Baldry, *The Battle against Heart Disease* (Cambridge, England: Cambridge University Press, 1971), pp. 174–75; and Richard J. Bing, ed., *Cardiology: The Evolution of the Science and the Art*, 2nd ed. (New Brunswick, N.J.: Rutgers University Press, 1999), pp. 14–26.

24. E. Nagourney, "Plumbing the Hearts of Siblings," *New York Times*, March 4, 2003, sec. F, p. 6, col. 1.

25. A. A. Panuju et al., "Is This Patient Having a Myocardial Infarction?" *Journal of the American Medical Association* 280 (1998): 1256–63; J. Chambers and C. Bass, "Atypical Chest Pain: Looking Beyond the Heart," *QJM: Monthly Journal of the Association of Physicians* 91 (March 1998): 239–44.

26. J. M. Gore et al., "The Increasing Use of Diagnostic Procedures in Patients with Acute Myocardial Infarction: A Community-Wide Perspective," in *Trends in Coronary Heart Disease Mortality: The Influence of Medical Care*, ed. Millicent W. Higgins and Russell V. Luepker (New York: Oxford University Press, 1988), p. 64.

27. M. M. G. Hunink et al., "The Recent Decline in Mortality from Coronary Heart Disease, 1980–1990: The Effect of Secular Trends in Risk Factors and Treatment," *Journal of the American Medical Association* 277 (1997): 540.

28. D. E. Nelson et al., "State Trends in Health Risk Factors and Receipt of Clinical Preventive Services among US Adults during the 1990s," *Journal of the American Medical Association* 287 (2002): 2659–67.

29. J. Stamler, "The Marked Decline in Coronary Heart Disease Mortality Rates in the United States, 1968–1981: Summary of Findings and Possible Explanations," *Cardiology* 72, no. 1–2 (1985): 11–22.

30. L. Goldman and E. F. Cook, "Reasons for the Decline in Coronary Heart Disease Mortality: Medical Interventions versus Life-Style Changes," in *Trends in Coronary Heart Disease Mortality: The Influence of Medical Care*, ed. Millicent W. Higgins and Russell V. Luepker (New York: Oxford University Press, 1988), p. 70.

31. P. G. McGovern et al., "Trends in Acute Coronary Heart Disease Mortality, Morbidity, and Medical Care from 1985 through 1997: The Minnesota Heart Study," *Circulation* 104 (2001): 19–24.

32. Nagourney, "Plumbing the Hearts of Siblings."

## CHAPTER 4: TREATMENT OF HEART DISEASE

1. Norman Cousins, *The Healing Heart: Antidotes to Panic and Helplessness* (New York: Norton, 1983), pp. 42–43.

2. Doris Kearns, *Lyndon Johnson and the American Dream* (New York: Harper and Row, 1976), p. 125.

3. I. Rosenfeld, "Why Cardiac Patients Can Take Heart," *Parade Magazine*, February 9, 2003, p. 8.

4. Rosenfeld, "Why Cardiac Patients Can Take Heart," p. 8.

5. Kathleen Berra et al., *Heart Attack: Advice for Patients by Patients* (New Haven: Yale University Press, 2002), pp. 34–51.

6. Berra, *Heart Attack,* pp. 67–75.

7. Berra, *Heart Attack,* p. 74.

8. The discussion on heart medications relies on several sources: National Heart, Lung, and Blood Institute, "Heart Disease and Medications," National Institutes of Health, http://www.nhlbi.nih.gov/actintime/hdm/hdm.htm (accessed April 2003); Bernard J. Gersh, ed., *Mayo Clinic Heart Book,* 2nd ed. (New York: William Morrow, 2000); Leonard S. Lilly, ed., *Pathophysiology of Heart Disease* (Baltimore, Md.: Lippincott, Williams, and Wilkins, 2003), pp. 371–422; and American Heart Association, *Heart Attack: Treatment, Recovery, Prevention* (New York: Random House, 1996), pp. 60–85.

9. Rosenfeld, "Why Cardiac Patients Can Take Heart," p. 10.

10. Consumer Education, "Aspirin for Reducing Your Risk of Heart Attack and Stroke: Know the Facts," U.S. Food and Drug Administration, http://www.fda.gov/cder/consumerinfo/dailyaspirin_brochure.htm (accessed April 2003).

11. Gersh, *Mayo Clinic Heart Book,* p. 297.

12. Steven Lehrer, *Explorers of the Body* (Garden City, N.Y.: Doubleday, 1979), pp. 14–21.

13. Lehrer, *Explorers of the Body,* p. 19.

14. Gersh, *Mayo Clinic Heart Book,* p. 298.

15. National Heart, Lung, and Blood Institute, "Types of Blood Pressure Medication," National Institutes of Health, http://www.nhlbi.nih.gov/hbp/treat/bpd_type.htm (accessed April 2003).

16. Gersh, *Mayo Clinic Heart Book,* p. 358.

17. Gersh, *Mayo Clinic Heart Book,* p. 298.

18. M. Meyer, "Is This the Drug for You," *AARP Bulletin,* November 2002, pp. 20–21.

19. S. J. Landers, "Beyond Cholesterol: New Uses for Statins," *American Medical News,* June 18, 2001, http://www/ama-assn.org/sci-pubs/amnews/pick_01/hlsb0618.htm.

20. R. A. Rosenblatt, "Clinton's Checkup Marred by Higher Cholesterol, Possible Skin Cancer," *Los Angeles Times,* January 13, 2001, p. A8.

21. P. R. Herbert, "Cholesterol Lowering with Statin Drugs, Risk of Stroke, and Total Mortality: An Overview of Randomized Trials." *Journal of the American Medical Association* 278 (1997): 313.

22. J. C. LaRosa, J. He, and S. Vuputuri, "Effect of Statins on Risk of Coronary Disease: A Meta-Analysis of Randomized Controlled Trials," *Journal of the American Medical Association* 282 (1999): 3240.

23. Herbert, "Cholesterol Lowering with Statin Drugs"; LaRosa, He, and Vuputuri, "Effect of Statins on Risk of Coronary Disease."

24. Meyer, "Is This the Drug for You," p. 20.

25. M. Mitka, "Cardiologists Like Statins—More Than Patients Do." *Journal of the American Medical Association* 286 (2001): 2799.

26. Landers, "Beyond Cholesterol."

27. Meyer, "Is This the Drug for You," p. 21.

28. Meyer, "Is This the Drug for You," p. 20.

29. Associated Press, "Cholesterol-Cutting Drugs Go Unused," *New York Times,* March 9, 1999, sec. F, p. 12, col. 1.

30. Meyer, "Is This the Drug for You," p. 21.

31. Mitka, "Cardiologists Like Statins," p. 2799.

32. J. Lindemuth, "Stand by Your Statins?" *AARP Bulletin*, May/June 2003, p. 18.

33. P. D. Thompson, P. Clarkson, and R. H. Karas, "Statin-Associated Myopathy," *Journal of the American Medical Association* 289 (2003): 1681–90.

34. D. A. Shaywitz and D. A. Ausiello, "Discovery: What Does the Unfolding Nature of the Statins Tell Us about the Nature of Medical Breakthroughs?" *Harvard Medical Alumni Bulletin*, Summer 2001, http://www.pasteur.harvard.edu/zones/Publications/articles/hmb_summer2001.htm.

35. Nobel Assembly at Karolinska, "The 1985 Nobel Prize in Physiology or Medicine," *Nobel e-Museum*, October 14, 1985, http://www.nobel.se/medicine/laureates/1985/press.html.

36. Richard J. Bing, ed., *Cardiology: The Evolution of the Science and the Art*, 2nd ed. (New Brunswick, N.J.: Rutgers University Press, 1999), p. 129.

37. National Heart, Lung, and Blood Institute, "Cholesterol Lowering Medicines," National Institutes of Health, http://www.nhlbi.nih.gov/chd/meds.htm (accessed April 2003).

38. Quoted in B. Fenley, "Trail of Discovery: How One Breakthrough Begets a Chain of Others," The University of Texas Southwestern Medical Center at Dallas, http://www3.utsouthwestern.edu/library/speccol/archives/nobel/trail_of_discovery1.htm (accessed April 2003).

39. "Michael S. Brown—Biography," *Nobel e-Museum*, June 18, 2002, http://www.nobel.se/medicine/laureates/1985/brown-bio.html.

40. "Joseph L. Goldstein—Biography," *Nobel e-Museum*, March 6, 2003, http://www.nobel.se/medicine/laureates/1985/goldstein-bio.html.

41. Gersh, *Mayo Clinic Heart Book*, p. 318.

42. American Heart Association, "Stent Procedure," *Heart and Stroke Encyclopedia*, http://www.americanheart.org/presenter.jhtml?identifier=4721 (accessed April 2003).

43. M. W. Cleman, "Coronary Angioplasty and Interventional Cardiology," in *Yale University School of Medicine Heart Book*, ed. Barry L. Zaret, Marvin Moser, and Lawrence S. Cohen, 1992, pp. 305–11, http://info.yale.edu/library/heartbk.

44. Rosenfeld, "Why Cardiac Patients Can Take Heart," p. 8.

45. Cleman, "Coronary Angioplasty and Interventional Cardiology."

46. Gersh, *Mayo Clinic Heart Book*, p. 322.

47. Gersh, *Mayo Clinic Heart Book*, p. 337–38.

48. L. Goldman and E. F. Cook, "Reasons for the Decline in Coronary Heart Disease Mortality: Medical Interventions versus Life-Style Changes," in *Trends in Coronary Heart Disease Mortality: The Influence of Medical Care*, ed. Millicent W. Higgins and Russell V. Luepker (New York: Oxford University Press, 1988), p. 70.

49. M. M. G. Hunink et al., "The Recent Decline in Mortality from Coronary Heart Disease, 1980–1990: The Effect of Secular Trends in Risk Factors and Treatment," *Journal of the American Medical Association* 277 (1997): 540.

50. Stanford University Medical Center, "Stanford Research Shows Medications Underused in Treating Heart Disease," News Release, January 1, 2003, http://stanfordhospital.com/newsEvents/newsReleases/2003/01/heartMedications.html.

51. P. G. McGovern et al., "Trends in Acute Coronary Heart Disease Mortality, Morbidity, and Medical Care from 1985 through 1997: The Minnesota Heart Study," *Circulation* 104 (2001): 19–24.

52. Cleman, "Coronary Angioplasty and Interventional Cardiology."

53. McGovern et al., "Trends in Acute Coronary Heart Disease Mortality."

54. W. D. Rosamond et al., "Trends in the Incidence of Myocardial Infarction and in Mortality Due to Coronary Heart Disease, 1987 to 1994," *New England Journal of Medicine* 339 (1998): 861–67.

55. G. Erikssen et al., "Hypothesis: The Recent Decline in Coronary Heart Disease Mortality—Mainly a Shift from Fatal to Non-Fatal Events?" *Scandinavian Cardiovascular Journal* 34 (October 2000): 468–74.

56. J. K. Borchardt, "New Technology Reduces the Profitability for New Drugs," *Scientist*, April 11, 2001, http://www.biomedcentral.com/news/200104/04.

57. Stanford University Medical Center, "Stanford Research Shows Medications Underused."

58. C. Lenfant, "Trends in Hypertension," *NIH Update*, April 21, 1999, http://www.nhlbi.nih.gov/new/press/hlbi21–9.htm.

## CHAPTER 5: SURGICAL TREATMENTS

1. Larry King, *Mr. King, You're Having a Heart Attack: How a Heart Attack and By-Pass Surgery Changed My Life* (New York: Delacorte Press, 1989).

2. Eugene Braunwald, ed., *Heart Disease: A Textbook of Cardiovascular Medicine* (Philadelphia: Saunders, 1997), p. 1316.

3. Centers for Disease Control and Prevention, "Table 9. Number of Ambulatory and Inpatient Procedures by Procedure Category and Location: United States, 1996," http://www.cdc.gov/nchswww/data/sr13_139.pdf (accessed October 2002); American Heart Association, "Open Heart Surgery Statistics," http://americanheart.org/presenter.jhtml?identifier=4674 (accessed October 2002).

4. American Heart Association, "Open Heart Surgery Statistics."

5. For overviews, see American Heart Association, "Bypass Surgery, Coronary Artery," http://americanheart.org/presenter.jhtml?identifier=4484 (accessed October 2002); and Cable News Network, "Heart Bypass Surgery Explained," November 5, 1996, http://www.cnn.com/WORLD/9611/05/yeltsin.bypass.

6. M. M. Levinson, "Coronary Artery Bypass Surgery," Heart Surgery Forum, http://www.hsforum.com/stories/storyReader$1482 (accessed October 2002).

7. P. E. Baldry, *The Battle against Heart Disease* (Cambridge, England: Cambridge University Press, 1971), pp. 167–68.

8. Baldry, *Battle against Heart Disease*, pp. 172–73.

9. National Library of Medicine, "Finding Aid to the John H. Gibbon Papers, 1903–1956: Biographical Note," http://www.nlm.gov/hmd/manuscripts/ead/gibbon.html (accessed January 2003).

10. National Library of Medicine, "Finding Aid to the John H. Gibbon Papers."

11. K. M. Scandrick, "Heart Valve Replacement," *Gale Encyclopedia of Medicine*, vol. 3, ed. Jacqueline L. Longe (Farmington Hills, Mich.: Gale Group, 2002), pp. 1550–52; P. A. Ford-Martin, "Heart Valve Repair," *Gale Encyclopedia of Medicine*, vol. 3 (2002), pp. 1549–50.

12. National Heart, Lung, and Blood Institute, "Facts about Heart and Heart-

Lung Transplants," http://www.nhlbi.nih.gov/health/public/heart/other/hrt_lung.htm (accessed October 2002).

13. British Broadcasting News, "Christian Barnard: Single-Minded Surgeon," September 2, 2001, http://news.bbc.co.uk/1/hi/health/1470356.stm.

14. British Broadcasting News, "Christian Barnard."

15. L. De Milto, "Heart Bypass Surgery," *Gale Encyclopedia of Medicine,* vol. 2, ed. Jacqueline L. Longe (Farmington Hills, Mich.: Gale Group, 2002), pp. 925–28.

16. Braunwald, *Heart Disease,* p. 1324.

17. Braunwald, *Heart Disease,* p. 1325.

18. Braunwald, *Heart Disease,* p. 1324.

19. Braunwald, *Heart Disease,* p. 1318.

20. E. J. Topol, "Aspirin with Bypass Surgery: From Taboo to New Standard of Care," *New England Journal of Medicine* 347 (2002): 1359–60.

21. T. B. Ferguson et al., "A Decade of Change: Risk Profiles and Outcomes for Isolated Coronary Artery Bypass Grafting Procedures, 1990–1999," *Annals of Thoracic Surgery* 73 (February 2002): 480–89.

22. Ferguson et al., "Decade of Change," p. 480.

23. Ferguson et al., "Decade of Change," p. 480.

24. National Institutes of Health, "Bypass Surgery and Angioplasty Equally Safe for Women and Men, Finds New Study," News Release, September 28, 1998, http://www.nhlbi.nih.gov/new/press/nhlbi-28.htm.

25. Braunwald, *Heart Disease,* pp. 1325–26.

26. C. M. Winslow et al., "The Appropriateness of Performing Coronary Artery Bypass Surgery," *Journal of the American Medical Association* 260 (1998): 505–9.

27. J. V. Tu et al., "Use of Cardiac Procedures and Outcomes in Elderly Patients with Myocardial Infarction in the United States and Canada," *New England Journal of Medicine* 336 (1997): 1500.

28. A. Bauman, "Too Many Bypasses?" *Men's Health* 13 (March 1998): 78–80.

29. H. M. Krumholz, "Cardiac Procedures, Outcomes, and Accountability," *New England Journal of Medicine* 336 (1997): 1521–23.

30. De Milto, "Heart Bypass Surgery."

31. A. C. Anyanwu and T. Treasure, "Unrealistic Expectations Arising from Mortality Data Reported in the Cardiothoracic Journals," *Journal of Thoracic and Cardiovascular Surgery* 123 (January 2002): 16–20.

32. O. A. Selnes and G. M. McKhann, "Coronary-Artery Bypass Surgery and the Brain," *New England Journal of Medicine* 344 (2001): 451–52.

33. M. F. Newman et al., "Longitudinal Assessment of Neurocognitive Function after Coronary-Artery Bypass Surgery," *New England Journal of Medicine* 344 (2001): 395–402.

34. D. B. Mark and M. F. Newman, "Protecting the Brain in Coronary Artery Bypass Graft Surgery," *Journal of the American Medical Association* 287 (2002): 1448–50.

35. R. H. Epstein, "Facing Up to Depression after a Bypass," *New York Times,* November 27, 2001, sec. F, p. 8, col. 1.

36. L. Goldman and E. F. Cook, "Reasons for the Decline in Coronary Heart Disease Mortality: Medical Interventions versus Life-Style Changes," in *Trends in Coronary Heart Disease Mortality: The Influence of Medical Care,* ed. Millicent W. Hig-

gins and Russell V. Luepker (New York: Oxford University Press, 1988), pp. 67–75.

37. T. Killip, "Has Coronary Artery Bypass Surgery Influenced Mortality from Cardiovascular Disease in the United States?" in *Trends in Coronary Heart Disease: The Influence of Medical Care*, ed. Millicent W. Higgins and Russell V. Luepker (New York: Oxford University Press, 1988), p. 257.

38. M. M. G. Hunink et al., "The Recent Decline in Mortality from Coronary Heart Disease, 1980–1990: The Effect of Secular Trends in Risk Factors and Treatment," *Journal of the American Medical Association* 277 (1997): 535–42.

39. B. Glenville, "Minimally Invasive Cardiac Surgery," *British Medical Journal* 319 (1999): 135–36.

40. Glenville, "Minimally Invasive Cardiac Surgery."

41. American Heart Association, "Minimally Invasive Heart Surgery," http://americanheart.org/presenter.jhtml?identifier=4702 (accessed October 2002).

## CHAPTER 6: TOBACCO USE

1. Iain Gately, *Tobacco: The Story of How Tobacco Seduced the World* (New York: Grove Press, 2001), p. 46.

2. Robert Sobel, *They Satisfy: the Cigarette in American Life* (Garden City, N.Y.: Anchor Books, 1978), pp. 50–51.

3. "Prevent Heart Disease," http://medicolegal.tripod.com/preventheart disease.htm (accessed March 2003).

4. Herbert H. Tidswell, *The Tobacco Habit: Its History and Pathology* (London: J. & A. Churchill, 1912).

5. Tidswell, *The Tobacco Habit*, pp. 64–65.

6. U.S. Department of Health, Education, and Welfare, *Smoking and Health: Report of the Advisory Committee to the Surgeon General of the Public Health Service* (Washington, D.C.: U.S. Department of Health, Education, and Welfare, 1964).

7. The figures are for the years 1982–1986 and come from U.S. Department of Health and Human Services, *Reducing the Health Consequences of Smoking: 25 Years of Progress—A Report of the Surgeon General* (Washington, D.C.: U.S. Department of Health and Human Services, 1989), pp. 150–51.

8. R. Doll et al., "Mortality in Relation to Smoking: 40 Years' Observations on Male British Doctors," *British Medical Journal* 309 (1994): 901–11.

9. U.S. Department of Health and Human Services, *Reducing the Health Consequences of Smoking*, p. 156.

10. Centers for Disease Control and Prevention, "Annual Smoking-Attributable Mortality, Years of Potential Life Lost, and Economic Costs—United States, 1995–1999," *MMWR Weekly* 51 (2002): 300–303.

11. M. Shaw, R. Mitchell, and D. Dorling, "Time for a Smoke? One Cigarette Reduces Your Life by 11 Minutes," *British Medical Journal* 320 (2000): 53.

12. U.S. Department of Health and Human Services, *Reducing the Health Consequences of Smoking*, p. 59.

13. U.S. Department of Health and Human Services, *Women and Smoking: A Report of the Surgeon General* (Washington, D.C.: U.S. Department of Health and Human Services, 2001), p. 237.

14. National Cancer Institute, *Risks Associated with Smoking Cigarettes with Low*

*Machine-Measured Yields of Tar and Nicotine,* Smoking and Tobacco Control Monograph 13 (Washington, D.C.: U.S. Department of Health and Human Services, 2001), p. 104.

15. C. Iribarren et al., "Effect of Cigar Smoking on the Risk of Cardiovascular Disease, Chronic Obstructive Pulmonary Disease, and Cancer in Men," *New England Journal of Medicine* 340 (1999): 1773–80.

16. G. Bolinder et al., "Smokeless Tobacco Use and Increased Cardiovascular Mortality among Swedish Construction Workers," *American Journal of Public Health* 84 (1994): 399–404.

17. National Cancer Institute, *Health Effects of Exposure to Environmental Tobacco Smoke: The Report of the California Environmental Protection Agency,* Smoking and Tobacco Control Monograph 10 (Washington, D.C.: U.S. Department of Health and Human Services, 1999), p. ES-4.

18. J. He et al., "Passive Smoking and the Risk of Coronary Heart Disease: A Meta-Analysis of Epidemiological Studies," *New England Journal of Medicine* 340 (1999): 920–26.

19. I. Kawachi et al., "A Prospective Study of Passive Smoking and Coronary Heart Disease," *Circulation* 95 (1997): 2374–79.

20. R. Otsuka, "Acute Effects of Passive Smoking on the Coronary Circulation in Healthy Young Adults," *Journal of the American Medical Association* 286 (2001): 436–41.

21. S. A. Glantz and W. W. Parmley, "Even a Little Secondhand Smoke Is Dangerous," *Journal of the American Medical Association* 286 (2001): 462–63.

22. M. D. Eisner et al., "Bartenders' Respiratory Health after Establishment of Smoke-Free Bars and Taverns," *Journal of the American Medical Association* 280 (1998): 1909–14.

23. See Jacob Sullum, *For Your Own Good: The Anti-Smoking Crusade and the Tyranny of Public Health* (New York: Free Press, 1998).

24. Although studies differ in conclusions, a review suggests that those finding little harm of smoking tend to be authored by those associated with the tobacco industry. See D. E. Barnes and L. A. Bero, "Why Review Articles on the Health Effects of Passive Smoking Reach Different Conclusions," *Journal of the American Medical Association* 279 (1998): 1566–70.

25. Edward L. Koven, *The Story behind the Haze* (Commack, N.Y.: Kroshka Books, 1998), pp. 37–64.

26. AMC Cancer Research Center, "Tobacco Use," http://www.amc.org/html/info/h_info_tobacco.html (accessed March 2003).

27. The discussion in this section relies on Eugene Braunwald, ed., *Heart Disease: A Textbook of Cardiovascular Medicine* (Philadelphia: Saunders, 1997), pp. 1147–48, 1397–98; and U.S. Department of Health and Human Services, *The Health Benefits of Smoking Cessation: A Report of the Surgeon General* (Washington, D.C.: U.S. Department of Health and Human Services, 1990), pp. 191–97.

28. The progress of atherosclerosis is measured by the thickness of the cartoid artery with ultrasound. See G. Howard, "Cigarette Smoking and Progression of Atherosclerosis: The Atherosclerosis Risk in Communities (ARIC) Study," *Journal of the American Medical Association* 279 (1998): 119–24.

29. U.S. Department of Health and Human Services, *Health Benefits of Smoking Cessation,* p. 239.

30. Braunwald, *Heart Disease*, p. 1148.

31. Braunwald, *Heart Disease*, p. 1397; I. S. Ockene, "Cigarette Smoking, Cardiovascular Disease, and Stroke: A Statement for Healthcare Professionals from the American Heart Association," *Circulation* 96 (1997): 3243–47.

32. C. M. Fichtenberg and S. A. Glantz, "Association of the California Tobacco Control Program with Declines in Cigarette Consumption and Mortality from Heart Disease," *New England Journal of Medicine* 343 (2000): 1772–77.

33. J. M. Lightwood and S. A. Glantz, "Short-Term Economic and Health Benefits of Smoking Cessation," *Circulation* 96 (1997): 1089–96.

34. G. Merriam, "Doctors Claim Link to Drop in Heart Attacks to Helena Smoking Ban," Missouilian.Com, April 2, 2003, http://www.missoulian.com/articles/2003/04/02/news/mtregional/news05.prt; and P. Peck, "Smoking Ban Saves Lives in Montana Town," WebMD, April 1, 2003, http://webmd.lycos.com/content/article/63/7/71871.htm.

35. U.S. Department of Health and Human Services, *The Health Consequences of Smoking: Nicotine Addiction. A Report of the Surgeon General* (Washington, D.C.: U.S. Department of Health and Human Services, 1988), pp. iv–v.

36. U.S. Department of Health and Human Services, *Reducing Tobacco Use: A Report of the Surgeon General* (Washington, D.C.: U.S. Department of Health and Human Services, 2000), p. 100.

37. U.S. Department of Health and Human Services, *Reducing the Health Consequences of Smoking*, p. 11.

38. U.S. Department of Health and Human Services, *Women and Smoking*, pp. 36–37.

39. U.S. Department of Health and Human Services, *Women and Smoking*, pp. 52–53, 60.

40. D. Satcher, "Cigars and Public Health," *New England Journal of Medicine* 340 (1999): 1829–31.

41. U.S. Department of Health and Human Services, *Reducing Tobacco Use*, p. 22.

42. American Lung Association, " 'There's Something about Mary' That Wasn't Funny—Cigarettes." American Lung Association State of the Air 2002, http://www.lungusa.org/press/association/aboutmary.htm (accessed April 2003).

43. J. D. Sargent et al., "Brand Appearances in Contemporary Cinema Films and Contribution to Global Marketing of Cigarettes," *Lancet* 357 (2002): 29–32.

44. American Lung Association, " 'There's Something about Mary' That Wasn't Funny."

45. L. K. Altman, "Heart Disease Progress Linked to Treatments," *New York Times*, February 19, 1997, sec. C, p. 8, col. 3.

46. J. Stamler, "The Marked Decline in Coronary Heart Disease Mortality Rates in the United States, 1968–1981: A Summary of Findings and Possible Explanations," *Cardiology* 72, no. 1–2 (1985): 11–22.

47. L. Goldman and E. F. Cook, "Reasons for the Decline in Coronary Heart Disease Mortality: Medical Interventions versus Life-Style Changes," in *Trends in Coronary Heart Disease Mortality: The Influence of Medical Care*, ed. Millicent W. Higgins and Russell V. Luepker (New York: Oxford University Press, 1988), pp. 67–75.

48. M. J. Thun et al., "Excess Mortality among Cigarette Smokers: Changes in a 20-Year Interval," *American Journal of Public Health* 85 (September 1995): 123–30.

49. M. M. G. Hunink et al., "The Recent Decline in Mortality from Coronary Heart Disease, 1980–1990: The Effect of Secular Trends in Risk Factors and Treatment," *Journal of the American Medical Association* 277 (1997): 535–42.

50. F. B. Hu et al., "Trends in the Incidence of Coronary Heart Disease and Changes in Diet and Lifestyle in Women," *New England Journal of Medicine* 343 (2000): 530–37.

51. A. Bitton, C. Fichtenberg, and S. A. Glantz, "Reducing Smoking Prevalence to 10% in Five Years," *Medical Student Journal of the American Medical Association* 286 (2001): 2733–34.

## CHAPTER 7: DIET AND EXERCISE

1. White House, "President Bush Launches HealthierUSA Initiative," Press Release, June 20, 2002, http://www.whitehouse.gov/news/releases/2002/06/20020620-6.html.

2. American Diabetes Association, "Basic Diabetes Information," http://www.diabetes.org (accessed March 2003).

3. Stephen Furst, *Confessions of a Couch Potato* (New York: McGraw-Hill, 2002).

4. D. Steinberg and A. M. Gotto, Jr., "Preventing Coronary Artery Disease by Lowering Cholesterol Levels," *Journal of the American Medical Association* 282 (1999): 2043–50.

5. Centers for Disease Control and Prevention, "Achievements in Public Health, 1900–1999: Decline in Deaths from Heart Disease and Stroke—United States, 1900–1999," *MMRW Weekly* 48, no. 30 (1999): 649–56.

6. Centers for Disease Control and Prevention, "Achievements in Public Health, 1900–1999."

7. D. Brown, "Keys of Nutrition," *Washington Post,* October 19, 2002, http://www.washingtonpost.com/ac2/wp-dyn?pagename = article&node = &contentId = A53532-2002Oct19.

8. J. W. Gofman, W. Young, and R. Tandy, "Ischemic Heart Disease, Atherosclerosis, and Longevity," *Circulation* 34 (October 1966): 679–97.

9. Steinberg and Gotto, "Preventing Coronary Artery Disease."

10. I. Hjermann et al., "Effect of Diet and Smoking Intervention on the Incidence of Coronary Heart Disease," *Lancet* 11 (1981): 1303–10.

11. The Lipid Research Clinic Group, "The Lipid Research Clinic's Coronary Primary Prevention Trial Results: II," *Journal of the American Medical Association* 251 (1984): 356–74.

12. J. M. McGinnis and W. H. Foege, "Actual Causes of Death in the United States," *Journal of the American Medical Association* 270 (1993): 2207–12.

13. American Heart Association, "American Heart Association Applauds Senate Appropriations Committee's Approval of HHS Budget for FY 2003," *Advocacy News,* July 22, 2002, http://www.americanheart.org/presenter.jhtml?identifier = 3003764.

14. "Ancel Keys," *MMWR Weekly* 48, no. 30 (1999): 651; Henry Blackburn, "Ancel Keys," University of Minnesota, http://mbbnet.umn.edu/blackburn_h.html (accessed March 2003); Brown, "Keys of Nutrition."

15. U.S. Food and Drug Administration, "Eating for a Healthy Heart," January 22, 2001, http://www.fda.gov/opacom/lowlit/hlyheart.html.

16. National Heart, Lung, and Blood Institute, "High Blood Cholesterol, What You Need to Know," National Cholesterol Education Program, http://www.nhlbi.nih.gov/health/public/heart/chol/hbc_what.htm (accessed March 2003).

17. American Heart Association, "Common Misconceptions about Cholesterol," http://www.americanheart.org/presenter.jhtml?identifier=3006030 (accessed March 2003).

18. National Heart, Lung, and Blood Institute, "High Blood Cholesterol."

19. Associated Press, "Study Questions Use of Nutrients in Heart Cases," *New York Times*, November 21, 2001, sec. A, p. 24, col. 4.

20. D. Grady, "More Support for Eating Fatty Fish," *New York Times*, April 10, 2002, sec. A, p. 22, col. 1.

21. P. Kris-Etherton et al., "New Guidelines Focus on Fish, Fish Oil, Omega-3 Fatty Acids," *Circulation* 106 (November 2002): 2747–57.

22. F. B. Hu and W. C. Willett, "Optimal Diets for Prevention of Coronary Heart Disease," *Journal of the American Medical Association* 288 (2002): 2569.

23. Associated Press, "Cutting Cholesterol with a Soy Diet," *New York Times*, March 18, 2003, sec. F, p. 7, col. 1.

24. R. Krauss et al., "AHA Dietary Guidelines, Revision 2000," *Stroke* 31 (November 2000): 2751–66.

25. M. Thun et al., "Alcohol Consumption and Mortality among Middle-Aged and Elderly U.S. Adults," *New England Journal of Medicine* 337 (1997): 1705–14.

26. A. Mokdad et al., "The Continuing Epidemics of Obesity and Diabetes in the United States," *Journal of the American Medical Association* 286 (2001): 1195–200.

27. American Heart Association, *Heart Disease and Stroke Statistics—2003 Update*, http://www.americanheart.org/presenter.jhtml?identifier=1928 (accessed May 2003), p. 28.

28. D. Ornish et al., "Intensive Lifestyle Changes for Reversal of Coronary Heart Disease," *Journal of the American Medical Association* 280 (1998): 2001–7. Popular books recommending an extremely low-fat diet include Dean Ornish, *Dr. Dean Ornish's Program for Reversing Heart Disease* (New York: Random House, 1990); and Robert Pritikin, *The New Pritikin Program* (New York: Simon and Schuster, 1990).

29. J. M. Ordovas et al., "Dietary Fat Intake Determines the Effect of a Common Polymorphism in the Hepatic Lipase Gene Promoter on High Density Lipoprotein Metabolism," *Circulation* 106 (2002): 2315–21.

30. U.S. Department of Agriculture, "Food Pyramid," http://www.nalusda.gov/fnic/Fpyr/pyramid.gif (accessed March 2003).

31. E. Saltos, "The Food Pyramid-Food Label Connection," U.S. Department of Agriculture, http://www.fda.gov/fdac/special/foodlabel/pyramid.html (accessed March 2003).

32. M. Duenwald, "Two Studies Indicate Atkins Diet May Improve Heart Health," *New York Times*, May 22, 2003, sec. A, p. 20, col. 3.

33. American Heart Association, "Dietary Guidelines, Revision 2000," http://216.185.102.50/dietaryguidelines (accessed March 2003).

34. American Heart Association, *Heart Disease and Stroke Statistics—2003 Update*, p. 34.

35. American Heart Association, *Heart Disease and Stroke Statistics—2003 Update,* p. 30.

36. American Heart Association, *Heart Disease and Stroke Statistics—2003 Update,* p. 30.

37. R. Cooper et al., "Trends and Disparities in Coronary Heart Disease, Stroke, and Other Cardiovascular Diseases in the United States: Findings of the National Conference on Cardiovascular Disease Prevention," *Circulation* 102 (2000): 3137–47.

38. American Heart Association, *Heart Disease and Stroke Statistics—2003 Update,* p. 30.

39. "Hey Buddy, Got an Hour?" *Washington Post,* September 17, 2002, p. F02.

40. J. O'Neil, "Regimen: Exercising to Your Own Rules," *New York Times,* February 18, 2003, sec. F, p. 6, col. 1.

41. M. Tanasescu et al., "Exercise Type and Intensity in Relation to Coronary Heart Disease in Men," *Journal of the American Medical Association* 288 (2002): 1994–2000.

42. American Heart Association, *Heart Disease and Stroke Statistics—2003 Update,* p. 32.

43. Obesity Education Initiative, "Guidelines on Overweight and Obesity: Electronic Textbook," http://www.nhlbi.nih.gov/guidelines/obesity/e_txtbk/ratnl/20.htm (accessed March 2003).

44. White House, "President Bush Launches HealthierUSA Initiative."

45. National Institutes of Health, "Health Implications of Obesity," *NIH Consensus Statement,* February 11–13, 1985.

46. For more information on the initiative, see U.S. Department of Health and Human Services, "Healthy People," http://www.healthypeople.gov (accessed March 2003).

47. McGinnis and Foege, "Actual Causes of Death in the United States."

48. S. Kenchaiah et al., "Obesity and the Risk of Heart Failure," *New England Journal of Medicine* 347 (2002): 305–13.

49. American Heart Association, *Heart Disease and Stroke Statistics—2003 Update,* p. 32.

50. A. Mokdad, "Prevalence of Obesity, Diabetes, and Obesity-Related Health Risk Factors, 2001," *Journal of American Medical Association* 289 (2003): 76–79.

51. American Heart Association, *Heart Disease and Stroke Statistics—2003 Update,* p. 35.

52. American Heart Association, *Heart Disease and Stroke Statistics—2003 Update,* p. 32; American Obesity Association, "Obesity in the U.S.," http://www.obesity.org/subs/fastfacts/obesity_US.shtml (accessed March 2003); K. Flegal et al., "Prevalence and Trends in Obesity among US Adults, 1999–2000," *Journal of the American Medical Association* 288 (2002): 1723–27.

53. American Heart Association, *Heart Disease and Stroke Statistics—2003 Update,* p. 34; Mokdad, "Prevalence of Obesity," pp. 76–79.

54. American Heart Association, *Heart Disease and Stroke Statistics—2003 Update,* p. 35.

55. American Heart Association, *Heart Disease and Stroke Statistics—2003 Update,* p. 36.

56. Steinberg and Gotto, "Preventing Coronary Artery Disease." The 1988–1994 figures come from NHANES III survey, the most recent statistics available.

57. American Heart Association, *Heart Disease and Stroke Statistics—2003 Update,* p. 36.

58. American Heart Association, *Heart Disease and Stroke Statistics—2003 Update,* pp. 30, 32, 36.

## CHAPTER 8: STRESS AND PSYCHOLOGICAL FACTORS

1. S. Canella, "Kile Found Dead in Chicago Hotel Room," SI.com, June 22, 2002, http://www.sportsillustratedcnn.com/baseball/news/2002/06/22/cards_kile_ap; Norwalk Radiology and Mammography Center, "Early Detection Exam for Heart Disease," July 3, 2002, http://www.norwalkradiology.com/news2.html.

2. British Heart Foundation, "British Heart Foundation Statistics Database 2003," *Coronary Heart Disease Statistics,* January 27, 2003, http://www.heartstats.org/datapage.asp?id=1652.

3. Meyer Friedman and Diane Ulmer, *Treating Type A Behavior—and Your Heart* (New York: Knopf, 1984), pp. 25–26.

4. Department of Internal Medicine, University of Iowa Virtual Hospital, "Stress and Your Heart: Facts and Statistics," *Iowa CHAMPS: Cardiac Rehabilitation Guide,* June 4, 2002, http://www.vh.org/adult/patient/internalmedicine/champs/stats.html.

5. Friedman and Ulmer, *Treating Type A Behavior,* pp. 9–43.

6. American Heart Association, "Stress and Heart Disease," http://www.americanheart.org/presenter.jhtml?identifier=4750 (accessed April 2003).

7. National Institutes of Health, "Stress System Malfunction Could Lead to Serious, Life Threatening Disease," September 9, 2002, http://www.nichd.nih.gov/new/releases/stress.cfm.

8. D. Krantz et al., "Effects of Mental Stress in Patients with Coronary Artery Disease: Evidence and Clinical Implications," *Journal of the American Medical Association* 283 (2000): 1800–1802.

9. Redford Williams and Virginia Williams, *Anger Kills* (New York: Times Books, 1993), p. 52.

10. National Institutes of Health, "Stress System Malfunction."

11. Department of Internal Medicine, University of Iowa Virtual Hospital, "Stress and Your Heart."

12. A. Rozanski, J. A. Blumenthal, and J. Kaplan, "Impact of Psychological Factors on the Pathogenesis of Cardiovascular Disease and Implications for Therapy," *Circulation* 99 (1999): 2192–2217.

13. American Heart Association, *Your Heart: An Owner's Manual* (Englewood Cliffs, N.J.: Prentice-Hall, 1995), p. 229; Williams and Williams, *Anger Kills,* pp. xiii–xv, 27–60.

14. A. H. Glassman and P. A. Shapiro, "Depression and the Course of Coronary Artery Disease," *American Journal of Psychiatry* 155 (January 1998): 4–11.

15. Glassman and Shapiro, "Depression and the Course of Coronary Artery Disease."

16. Krantz, "Effects of Mental Stress."

17. L. E. Spieker et al., "Mental Stress Induces Prolonged Endothelial Dysfunc-

tion via Endothelin-A Receptors," *Circulation* 105 (2002): 2817–20; American Heart Association, "Stress Leaves Blood Vessels Tightly Wound," Journal Report, http://www.americanheart.org/presenter.jhtml?identifier=3002753 (accessed April 2003).

18. H. Iso et al., "Perceived Mental Stress and Mortality from Cardiovascular Disease among Japanese Men and Women," *Circulation* 106 (2002): 1229–36; American Heart Association, "High Mental Stress Linked with Increased Risk of Cardiovascular Death," Journal Report, August 7, 2002, http://www.americanheart.org/presenter.jhtml?identifier=3004252.

19. American Heart Association, "Triggers for Sudden Cardiac Arrest Differ by Gender," Meeting Report, April 24, 2002,http://www.americanheart.org/presenter.jhtml?identifier=3002347.

20. L. R. Wulsin and B. M. Singal, "Do Depressive Symptoms Increase the Risk for the Onset of Coronary Disease? A Systematic Quantitative Review," *Psychosomatic Medicine* 65 (March–April 2003): 201–10.

21. National Institute of Mental Health, "Depression Can Break Your Heart," NIH Publication No. 01-4592, January 2001, http://www.nimh.nih.gov/publicat/heartbreak.pdf.

22. Krantz, "Effects of Mental Stress."

23. National Institute of Mental Health, "Depression Can Break Your Heart."

24. Associated Press, "Pessimism Can Be Deadly for Heart Patients," *New York Times*, April 16, 1994, sec. 1, p. 8, col. 2.

25. National Institute of Mental Health, "Depression Can Break Your Heart."

26. National Institutes of Health, "Stress System Malfunction Could Lead to Serious, Life Threatening Disease," September 9, 2002, http://www.nichd.nih.gov/new/releases/stress.cfm.

27. National Institute of Mental Health, "Depression Can Break Your Heart"; R. C. Ziegelstein et al., "Patients with Depression Are Less Likely to Follow Recommendations to Reduce Cardiac Risk during Recovery from a Myocardial Infarction," *Archives of Internal Medicine* 160 (2000): 1818–23.

28. B. W. Penninx et al., "Depression and Cardiac Mortality: Results from a Community-Based Longitudinal Study," *Archives of General Psychiatry* 58 (March 2001): 221–27.

29. F. Lespérance et al., "Five-Year Risk of Cardiac Mortality in Relation to Initial Severity and One-Year Changes in Depression Symptoms after Myocardial Infarction," *Circulation* 105 (2002): 1049–53.

30. Williams and Williams, *Anger Kills*, p. xiv.

31. E. Nagourney, "At Risk: Blow a Gasket, for Your Heart," *New York Times*, February 11, 2003, sec. F, p. 6, col. 1.

32. Friedman and Ulmer, *Treating Type A Behavior*, pp. 13–15.

33. Krantz, "Effects of Mental Stress."

34. Williams and Williams, *Anger Kills*, pp. xv, 47, 48, 54–56.

35. Associated Press, "Pessimism Can Be Deadly."

36. P. P. Chang, "Anger in Young Men and Subsequent Premature Cardiovascular Disease," *Archives of Internal Medicine* 162 (2002): 901–6; C. Iribarren et al., "Association of Hostility with Coronary Artery Calcification in Young Adults," *Journal of the American Medical Association* 283 (2000): 2546–51.

37. Associated Press, "Pessimism Can Be Deadly."

38. American Heart Association, *Your Heart: An Owner's Manual*, pp. 227–42.

39. British Heart Foundation, "Psychosocial Well-Being," British Heart Foundation Statistics Database 2002, http://www.dphpc.ox.ac.uk/bhfhprg/2000/2002/pyschosocialwellbeing.html (accessed April 2003).

40. K. M. MacMahon and G. Y. Lip, "Psychological Factors in Heart Failure," *Archives of Internal Medicine* 162 (2002): 509–16.

41. N. Frasure-Smith et al., "Social Support, Depression, and Mortality during the First Year after Myocardial Infarction," Circulation 101 (2000): 1919–24.

42. Krantz, "Effects of Mental Stress."

43. Krantz, "Effects of Mental Stress."

44. British Heart Foundation, "Psychosocial Well-Being."

45. National Institutes of Health, "Stress System Malfunction," http://www.nichd.nih.gov/new/releases/stress.cfm.

46. W. A. Karlin, E. Brondolo, and J. Schwartz, "Workplace Social Support and Ambulatory Cardiovascular Activity in New York City Traffic Agents," *Psychosomatic Medicine* 65 (March–April 2003): 167–76.

47. British Heart Foundation, "Psychosocial Well-Being."

48. K. Orth-Gomér et al., "Marital Stress Worsens Prognosis in Women with Coronary Heart Disease: The Stockholm Female Coronary Risk Study," *Journal of the American Medical Association* 284 (2000): 3008–14.

49. K. A. Mathews and B. B. Gump, "Chronic Work Stress and Marital Dissolution Increase Risk of Posttrial Mortality in Men from the Multiple Risk Factor Intervention Trial," *Archives of Internal Medicine* 162 (2002): 309–15.

50. National Institute of Mental Health, "Depression Can Break Your Heart."

51. Dean Ornish, *Dr. Dean Ornish's Program for Reversing Heart Disease* (New York: Random House, 1990).

52. Krantz, "Effects of Mental Stress."

53. British Heart Foundation, "British Heart Foundation Statistics Database 2003."

54. National Institute of Mental Health, "Depression Can Break Your Heart."

## CHAPTER 9: WOMEN AND HEART DISEASE

1. Kathleen Berra et al., *Heart Attack: Advice for Patients by Patients* (New Haven, Conn.: Yale University Press, 2002), pp. 102–11.

2. American Heart Association, *Heart Disease and Stroke Statistics—2003 Update*, http://www.americanheart.org/presenter.jhtml?identifier=1928 (accessed May 2003), p. 4.

3. American Heart Association, "Statistical Fact Sheet—Populations: Men and Cardiovascular Disease," http://www.americanheart.org/presenter.jhtml?identifier=2011 (accessed May 2003).

4. American Heart Association, "Statistical Fact Sheet—Populations: Women and Cardiovascular Disease," http://www.americanheart.org/presenter.jhtml?identifier=2011 (accessed May 2003).

5. American Heart Association, "Facts about Women and Cardiovascular Diseases," http://www.americanheart.org/presenter.jhtml?identifier=2876 (accessed May 2003).

6. American Heart Association, *Heart Disease and Stroke Statistics—2003 Update*, pp. 4, 6.

7. American Heart Association, "Women and Cardiovascular Diseases."

8. P. Lee et al., "Representation of Elderly Persons and Women in Published Randomized Trials of Acute Coronary Syndromes," *Journal of the American Medical Association* 286 (2001): 708–13; N. Wenger, "Exclusion of the Elderly and Women from Coronary Trials: Is Their Quality of Care Compromised?" *Journal of the American Medical Association* 268 (1992): 1460–61.

9. L. Mosca et al., "Guide to Preventive Cardiology for Women: AHA/ACC Scientific Statement: Consensus Panel Statement," *Circulation* 99 (1999): 2480–84.

10. Morris Notelovitz and Diana Tonnessen, *The Essential Heart Book for Women* (New York: St. Martin's Press, 1996), pp. 25–30.

11. Notelovitz and Tonnessen, *Essential Heart Book for Women*, pp. 28–30; B. Abramson, "Risk Factors and Primary Prevention of Ischemic Heart Disease in Women," *Canadian Journal of Cardiology* 17 (2001): 24D–31D.

12. American Heart Association, "Is It Gender Difference or Gender Bias," http://www.americanheart.org/presenter.jhltm?identifier = 2633 (accessed April 2003).

13. American Heart Association, "Is It Gender Difference or Gender Bias."

14. Mosca et al., "Guide to Preventive Cardiology for Women."

15. G. Kolata, "Hormone Studies: What Went Wrong?" *New York Times*, April 22, 2003, sec. F, p. 1.

16. V. Harden, "A Short History of the National Institutes of Health," http://www.nih.gov/od/museum/exhibits/history/index.html (accessed May 2003); National Institutes of Health, "NIH Guidelines on the Inclusion of Women and Minorities as Subjects in Clinical Research," August 2, 2000, http://grants.nih.gov/grants/guide/notice-files/NOT-OD-00-048.html.

17. Feminist Research Center, "Empowering Women in Medicine: What's Wrong with This Picture," Feminist Majority Foundation, http://www.feminist.org/research/ewm_toc.html (accessed May 2003).

18. Feminist Research Center, "Empowering Women in Medicine: The Feminine Difference." Feminist Majority Foundation, http://www.feminist.org/research/ewm_diff.html (accessed May 2003).

19. Feminist Research Center, "Empowering Women in Medicine: The National Medical Feminist Agenda," Feminist Majority Foundation, http://www.feminist.org/research/ewm_agen.html (accessed May 2003).

20. Notelovitz and Tonnessen, *Essential Heart Book for Women*, pp. 1–8.

21. Notelovitz and Tonnessen, *Essential Heart Book for Women*, p. 8.

22. Mosca et al., "Guide to Preventative Cardiology for Women."

23. Notelovitz and Tonnessen, *Essential Heart Book for Women*, pp. 25–28.

24. Notelovitz and Tonnessen, *Essential Heart Book for Women*, p. 27.

25. American Heart Association, "Women and Cardiovascular Diseases."

26. L. Mosca, "Cardiovascular Disease in Women," *Circulation* 96 (1997): 2468–82.

27. D. A. Lawlor, S. Ebrahim, and G. Davey Smith, "Sex Matters: Secular and Geographical Trends in Sex Differences in Coronary Heart Disease Mortality," *British Medical Journal* 323 (2001): 541–45.

28. American Heart Association, *Heart Disease and Stroke Statistics—2003 Update*, pp. 4, 6, 8.

29. American Heart Association, *Heart Disease and Stroke Statistics—2003 Update*, p. 11.

30. American Heart Association, "Women and Cardiovascular Diseases."

31. American Heart Association, *Heart Disease and Stroke Statistics—2003 Update*, p. 12.

32. American Heart Association, *Heart Disease and Stroke Statistics—2003 Update*, pp. 11, 13.

33. American Heart Association, *Heart Disease and Stroke Statistics—2003 Update*, pp. 12, 17.

34. American Heart Association, "Women and Cardiovascular Diseases."

35. American Heart Association, *Heart Disease and Stroke Statistics—2003 Update*, p. 5.

36. M. C. Petrie, et al., "Current Perspectives: Failure of Women's Hearts," *Circulation* 99 (1999): 2334–41.

37. American Heart Association, *Heart Disease and Stroke Statistics—2003 Update*, p. 23.

38. Petrie, "Current Perspectives: Failure of Women's Hearts."

39. T. Simon et al., "Sex Differences in the Prognosis of Congestive Heart Failure Results from the Cardiac Insufficiency Bisoprolol Study (CIBIS II)," *Circulation* 103 (2001): 375.

40. American Heart Association, "Women and Cardiovascular Diseases."

41. American Heart Association, *Heart Disease and Stroke Statistics—2003 Update*, p. 34.

42. Mosca et al., "Guide to Preventative Cardiology for Women."

43. British Heart Foundation, "British Heart Foundation Statistics Database 2003," *Coronary Heart Disease Statistics*, January 27, 2003, http://www.heartstats.org/datapage.asp?id = 1652.

44. Abramson, "Risk Factors and Primary Prevention," p. 27D.

45. A. M. Kanaya et al., "Explaining the Sex Difference in Coronary Heart Disease Mortality among Patients with Type 2 Diabetes Mellitus: A Meta-Analysis," *Archives of Internal Medicine* 162 (2002): 1737–45.

46. American Heart Association, "Women and Cardiovascular Diseases."

47. American Heart Association, "Women and Cardiovascular Diseases"; Mosca et al., "Guide to Preventative Cardiology for Women"; American Heart Association, *Heart Disease and Stroke Statistics—2003 Update*, p. 28.

48. American Heart Association, *Heart Disease and Stroke Statistics—2003 Update*, p. 30.

49. Abramson, "Risk Factors and Primary Prevention," p. 27D.

50. K. Orth-Gomér et al., "Marital Stress Worsens Prognosis in Women with Coronary Heart Disease: The Stockholm Female Coronary Risk Study," *Journal of the American Medical Association* 284 (2000): 3008–14; K. A. Mathews and B. B. Gump, "Chronic Work Stress and Marital Dissolution Increase Risk of Posttrial Mortality in Men from the Multiple Risk Factor Intervention Trial," *Archives of Internal Medicine* 162 (2002): 309–15.

51. Mosca, "Cardiovascular Disease in Women," pp. 2468–82.

## CHAPTER 10: TWENTIETH-CENTURY TRENDS

1. C. Lenfant, "Heart Research: Celebration and Renewal." National Heart, Lung, and Blood Institute, December 2, 1997, http://www.nhlbi.nih.gov/funding.fromdir/hrt_res.htm.

2. National Heart, Lung, and Blood Institute, "50 Years of Progress in Heart, Lung, and Blood Research: NHLBI Celebrates Its Golden Anniversary," *Heart Memo,* Fall 1997, pp. 1, 13–15.

3. C. Lenfant, "Letter from the Director," *Heart Memo,* Fall 1997, p. 2.

4. A. R. Omran, "Epidemiological Transition in the U.S.," *Population Bulletin* 32 (1977): 1–40.

5. J. H. Wolleswinkel-van den Bosch et al., "Mortality Decline in the Netherlands in the Period 1850–1992: A Turning Point Analysis," *Social Science and Medicine* 47 (August 1998): 429–43.

6. R. A. Stallones, "The Rise and Fall of Ischemic Heart Disease," *Scientific American* 243 (November 1980): 43–50.

7. W. E. Stehbens, "An Appraisal of the Epidemic Rise of Coronary Heart Disease and Its Decline," *Lancet* 1 (8533): 606–11.

8. Stallones, "Rise and Fall of Ischemic Heart Disease."

9. Stallones, "Rise and Fall of Ischemic Heart Disease."

10. Wolleswinkel-van den Bosch et al., "Mortality Decline in the Netherlands," pp. 429–43.

11. Stehbens, "Appraisal of the Epidemic Rise of Coronary Heart Disease."

12. Stehbens, "Appraisal of the Epidemic Rise of Coronary Heart Disease," p. 606.

13. Stallones, "Rise and Fall of Ischemic Heart Disease."

14. C. Lenfant, "Foreword," in *Trends in Coronary Heart Disease Mortality: The Influence of Medical Care,* ed. Millicent W. Higgins and Russell V. Luepker (New York: Oxford University Press, 1988), p. vi.

15. T. J. Thom and J. Maurer, "Time Trends for Coronary Heart Disease Mortality and Morbidity," in *Trends in Coronary Heart Disease Mortality: The Influence of Medical Care,* ed. Millicent W. Higgins and Russell V. Luepker (New York: Oxford University Press, 1988), pp. 7–15.

16. Thom and Maurer, "Time Trends for Coronary Heart Disease Mortality and Morbidity," pp. 7–15.

17. V. Harden, "A Short History of the National Institutes of Health," National Institutes of Health, http://www.nih.gov/od/museum/exhibits/history/index.html (accessed May 2003).

18. The figures for this section come from the following sources: National Center for Health Statistics, *International Mortality Data Base* (Washington, D.C.: U.S. Department of Health and Human Services, 1995); Centers for Disease Control and Prevention, "CDC Wonder," October 21, 1998, http://wonder.cdc.gov/.

19. Identifying these separate causes of death and recording them on death certificates can pose difficulties. Deaths that occur unexpectedly outside a hospital and do not involve an autopsy require a certain amount of guesswork to determine the cause. Errors inevitably result. In addition, selecting one primary or underlying cause of death from heart disease, although making for simplicity, may mask the full syndrome of problems and contribute to incompleteness and error in reporting. Still, even if not exact, the figures indicate in broad terms the prevalence of various types of heart disease.

20. E. Braunwald, "Cardiovascular Medicine at the Turn of the Millennium: Triumphs, Concerns, and Opportunities," *New England Journal of Medicine* 337 (1997): 1360–69.

21. L. Bonneux et al., "Estimating Clinical Morbidity Due to Ischemic Heart Disease and Congestive Heart Failure: The Future Rise of Heart Failure," *American Journal of Public Health* 84 (January 1994): 20–28.

22. R. Cooper et al., "Trends and Disparities in Coronary Heart Disease, Stroke, and Other Cardiovascular Diseases in the United States: Findings of the National Conference on Cardiovascular Disease Prevention," *Circulation* 102 (2000): 3137–47.

23. Cooper et al., "Trends and Disparities in Coronary Heart Disease," p. 3142.

24. R. O. Bonow et al., "The International Burden of Cardiovascular Disease: Responding to the Emerging Global Epidemic," *Circulation* 106 (2002): 1602–5.

25. National Heart, Lung, and Blood Institute, "Morbidity and Mortality: 2002 Chart Book on Cardiovascular, Lung, and Blood Diseases," http://www.nhlbi.nih.gov/resources/docs/02-chtbk.pdf (accessed October 2002), p. 24.

26. The listing relies on The Franklin Institute Online, "Milestones in Cardiology," http://sln.fi.edu/biosci/history/firsts.html (accessed January 2003); and H. S. L. Lee, ed., *Dates in Cardiology* (New York: Parthenon, 2000).

27. E. Barnett and J. Halverson, "Local Increases in Coronary Heart Disease Mortality among Blacks and Whites in the United States, 1985–1995," *American Journal of Public Health* 91 (September 2001): 1499–1506.

28. L. H. Kuller, "Commentary on Coronary Artery Disease in Blacks," *Public Health Reports* 110 (September/October 1995): 570–71.

29. Cooper et al., "Trends and Disparities in Coronary Heart Disease."

30. G. A. Kaplan and J. E. Keil, "Socioeconomic Factors and Cardiovascular Disease: A Review of the Literature," *Circulation* 88 (October 1993): 1973–98.

31. A. V. Diez Roux et al., "Neighborhood of Residence and Incidence of Coronary Heart Disease," *New England Journal of Medicine* 345 (2001): 99–106.

32. K. Steenland, J. Henley, and M. Thun, "All-Cause and Cause-Specific Death Rates by Educational Status for Two Million People in Two American Cancer Society Cohorts, 1959–1996," *American Journal of Epidemiology* 156 (2002): 11–21.

33. G. Pappas et al., "The Increasing Disparity in Mortality between Socioeconomic Groups in the United States, 1960 and 1986," *New England Journal of Medicine* 329 (1993): 103–9.

34. E. Barnett and J. Halverson, "Disparities in Premature Coronary Heart Disease Mortality by Region and Urbanicity among Black and White Adults Ages 35–64, 1985–1995," *Public Health Reports* 115 (January/February 2000): 52–64.

35. Cooper et al., "Trends and Disparities in Coronary Heart Disease."

36. M. L. Casper et al., *Women and Heart Disease: An Atlas of Racial and Ethnic Disparities in Mortality* (Morgantown, W.V.: Office for Social Environment and Health Research, West Virginia University, 1999).

37. Cooper et al., "Trends and Disparities in Coronary Heart Disease," p. 3139.

38. G. R. Najem, D. E. Hutcheon, and M. Feuerman, "Changing Patterns of Ischaemic Heart Disease Mortality in New Jersey 1968–1982, and the Relationship of Urbanization," *International Journal of Epidemiology* 19 (March 1990): 26–31.

39. The listing relies on The Franklin Institute Online, "Milestones in Cardiology"; and Lee, *Dates in Cardiology*.

40. F. Levi et al., "Trends in Mortality from Cardiovascular and Cerebrovascular Diseases in Europe and Other Areas of the World," *Heart* (August 2002): 119–24.

41. T. J. Thom, "International Mortality from Heart Disease: Rates and Trends," *International Journal of Epidemiology* 18 (1989): S20–S28.

42. Levi et al., "Trends in Mortality from Cardiovascular and Cerebrovascular Diseases."

43. C. J. Murray and A. D. Lopez, "Alternative Projections of Mortality and Disability by Cause 1990–2020: Global Burden of Disease Study," *Lancet* 349 (1997): 1498–1504.

44. Bonow et al., "International Burden of Cardiovascular Disease," pp. 1602–5.

45. F. C. Lampe et al., "Is the Prevalence of Coronary Heart Disease Falling in British Men?" *Heart* 86 (November 2001): 499–505.; W. D. Rosamond et al., "Coronary Heart Disease Trends in Four United States Communities: The Atherosclerosis Risk in Communities (ARIC) Study 1987–1996," *International Journal of Epidemiology* 30 (October 2001): S17–S22.

46. C. A. Derby et al., "Sex-Specific Trends in Validated Coronary Heart Disease Rates in Southeastern New England, 1980–1991," *American Journal of Epidemiology* 151 (2000): 417–29.

47. L. Bonneux, J. J. Barendregt, and P. J. van der Mass, "The New Old Epidemic of Coronary Heart Disease," *American Journal of Public Health* 89 (March 1999): 379–82.

48. Cooper et al., "Trends and Disparities in Coronary Heart Disease."

## CHAPTER 11: LOOKING AHEAD

1. M. Allen, "Cheney Says He'll Run for Reelection with Bush," *Washington Post*, May 8, 2003, http://www.washingtonpost.com/ac2/wp-dyn/A27568-2003May7.html.

2. Allen B. Weisse, *Heart to Heart: The Twentieth-Century Battle against Cardiac Disease* (New Brunswick, N.J.: Rutgers University Press, 2002), p. 349.

3. Weisse, *Heart to Heart*, p. 350.

4. The information in this section is based on American Heart Association, "American Heart Association's Top 10 Research Advances for 2002," December 31, 2002, http://www.americanheart.org/presenter.jhtml?identifier = 3007336; and American Heart Association, "American Heart Association's Top 10 Research Advances for 2001," December 31, 2001, http://www.americanheart.org/presenter.jhtml?identifier = 3000094.

5. American Heart Association, "American Heart Association's Top 10 Research Advances for 2002."

6. National Heart, Lung, and Blood Institute, "Strategic Plan FY 2003–2007: Treatment of Disease," http://www.nhlbi.nih.gov/resources/docs/plan/treat.htm (accessed May 2003).

7. C. Lenfant, "Fixing the Failing Heart," *Circulation*, February 18, 1997, http://www.nhlbi.gov/funding/fromdir/circ197.htm.

8. N. Wade, "Teaching the Body to Heal Itself," *New York Times*, November 7, 2000, http://www.nytimes.com/learning/general/featured_articles/001107tuesday.html.

9. M. Finley, "Anatomy of an Entrepreneur," *Masters Forum*, April 2, 2001,

http://www.mastersforum.com/archives/summaries2001/haseltine/haseltine-notes.htm; Alliance for Aging Research, "Regenerative Medicine: Paving the Way for a Healthier Old Age," *Living Longer,* Summer 2002, http://www.agingresearch.org/living_longer/summer00/printer_science.html; Life Extension Foundation, "Interview with William Haseltine," *Life Extension Magazine,* July 2002, http://www.lef.org/magazine/mag2002/jul2002_report_haseltine_02.html.

10. Alliance for Aging Research, "Regenerative Medicine."

11. P. Schwartz, "Regenerative Medicine Is the Future," *Red Herring,* October 1, 2001, http://www.redherring.com/mag/issues105/167518.html.

12. C. Semsarian, "Stem Cells in Cardiovascular Disease: From Cell Biology to Clinical Therapy," *Internal Medicine Journal* 32 (May–June 2002): 259.

13. "Interview with William Haseltine."

14. "Bill Haseltine," *Fortune,* June 25, 2001, http://linkage.rockefeller.edu/wli/reading/haseltine.html.

15. Schwartz, "Regenerative Medicine Is the Future."

16. Wade, "Teaching the Body to Heal Itself."

17. Human Genome Sciences, "Human Genome Sciences," Management Profiles, http://www.hgsi.com/cprofile/mgmt.html (accessed May 2003).

18. *E-Biomed: The Journal of Regenerative Medicine,* Mary Anne Liebert Publishers, http://liebertpub.com/ebi/default1.asp (accessed May 2003).

19. Human Genome Sciences, "Human Genome Sciences."

20. "Bill Haseltine."

21. "Interview with William Haseltine."

22. R. Cooper et al., "Trends and Disparities in Coronary Heart Disease, Stroke, and Other Cardiovascular Diseases in the United States: Findings of the National Conference on Cardiovascular Disease Prevention," *Circulation* 102 (2000): 3137–47.

23. Cooper et al., "Trends and Disparities in Coronary Heart Disease."

24. C. Connolly, "Health Costs of Obesity Near Those of Smoking," *Washington Post,* May 14, 2003, http://www.washingtonpost.com/ac2/wp-dyn/A51654-2003May13.htm.

25. Centers for Disease Control, "DATA2010: The Healthy People 2010 Database," http://www.cdc.gov/nchs/about/otheract/hpdata2010/abouthp.htm (accessed May 2003).

26. Connolly, "Health Costs of Obesity."

27. S. Squires, "New Guidelines Issued for High Blood Pressure," *Washington Post,* May 14, 2003, http://www.washingtonpost.com/ac2/wp-dyn/A54259-2003May14.htm.

28. Cooper et al., "Trends and Disparities in Coronary Heart Disease."

29. National Center for Complementary and Alternative Medicine, "What Is Complementary and Alternative Medicine?" October 21, 2001, http://nccam.nih.gov/health/whatiscam.

30. George Jacob, "Heart Infocenter," *Holistic-Online,* http://www.holistic-online.com/Remedies/Heart (accessed May 2003); Cardiac Yoga, "What Is Cardiac Yoga," http://www.cardiacyoga.com/home.html (accessed May 2003).

31. Hans R. Larsen, "Alternative Medicine: Why So Popular?" http://www.yourhealthbase.com/alternative_medicine.html (accessed May 2003).

32. Larsen, "Alternative Medicine."

33. National Institutes of Health, "National Center for Complementary and Alternative Medicine," http://www.nih.gov/about/almanac/organization/NCCAM.htm (accessed May 2003).

# Index

**About the Authors**

FRED C. PAMPEL is Professor of Sociology and Epidemiology Research Associate at the University of Colorado Institute of Behavioral Science Population Program. He has authored eight earlier books, including the *International Handbook of Old-Age Insurance* (Praeger, 1991).

SETH PAULEY is a copywriter for Facts on File in New York City and a freelance writer.